A Guide to

Waterless Cooking

and greaseless cooking for better health

Instruction, Nutrition,
Recipes and Weight
Management

Chef Charles Knight

ISBN: I-4392-2602-4
ISBN-I3: 9781439226025

Visit www.booksurge.com to order additional copies.

INTRODUCTION

The answer to better health is exercise and the food we eat. Nutritious, low-fat, low-sodium, and reduced carbohydrate meals, are fundamental to today's health-conscious lifestyles; meals that help reduce dangerous cholesterol cut unwanted calories and retain important minerals, vitamins, and life giving enzymes. All of our fresh foods have a built-in natural goodness. But the wonderful health-giving values you paid dearly for at your grocery store may soon disappear in your kitchen. With old-fashioned conventional cooking methods, fresh vegetables must be peeled, boiled, or steamed, and subjected to high heat, not to mention the use of cooking fats and oils and the extremely high temperatures of the microwave. All of this results in the irreplaceable loss of a large share of the vital minerals, vitamins and enzymes that we need for better health.

Waterless, greaseless food preparation creates wholesome, great tasting meals, without sacrificing vitamins, minerals and enzymes. Furthermore, the methods you will learn thoroughly capture the wonderful flavors we expect in our meals. It's possible because of this unique cooking method. Most foods cook on low or medium-low heat, below the boiling temperature, in a vapor seal. The vapor seal method of waterless cooking is the secret that retains vital nutritional values. By eliminating the need for peeling, boiling, steaming and microwaving, vegetables and fruits come to the table with a "garden fresh" taste, and meats are gently seared and browned and cooked in their own natural juices, without the need for high calorie oils and fat. It's a whole new experience in cooking and taste, and a key benefit for better health.

Because food preparation is easy and efficient, waterless, greaseless cooking has become the preferred method of millions of home cooks who are dedicated to better health through healthier cooking techniques. *A Guide to Waterless Cooking* contains exciting recipes that will bring nature's goodness to your table every day.

Two sound fundamentals are to always underscore anything we include in this cookbook. First, the recipes must be quick and easy to prepare, with ingredients that are readily available. And second, every recipe must be tasty and healthful.

Chef David Knight, President
Health Craft Cookware

TABLE OF CONTENTS

i   **INTRODUCTION**
      Chef David Knight

v   **FORWARD**
      Ann Hunter, PhD, RD, LD, FADA

1   **BASIC COOKWARE CARE**
      Cleaning Before First Use

3   **THE VAPOR SEAL METHOD**
      Waterless Cooking
      Cooking Meats without Grease
      Top-of-the-Range Baking
      Stack Cooking

9   **BASIC PRODUCT INFORMATION**
      Features to Consider
      Here's what to look for:
      Induction Cooking

13   **BASIC U.S./METRIC CONVERSIONS**

15   **RECIPE FEATURES**
      Nutritional Breakdown Explanation

17   **ADAPTING RECIPES**

19   **BASIC COOKING INSTRUCTIONS**
      Roasting Meats on-to-of-the Stove
      Pan Broiling Chicken, Steaks & Chops
      Testing Meat for Doneness
      Pan Frying
      Steaming & Braising Meats
      Waterless Cooking Fruits & Vegetables
      Cooking Pastas & Grains
      Pasta Dictionary & Grain Chart
      Cooking Eggs

33   **NUTRITION BASICS**
      Staying Fit with Health Craft – Daily Food Guide
      The American Cancer Society Recommendations
      Dietary Intake – Metabolism

41   **NUTRITION FACTS**
      Understanding and Using Food Labels

46 CALORIE POINT SYSTEM

  Calorie/Carbohydrate Point Conversions

  Calorie, Carbohydrate, Sodium Conversion Charts

  Sample Menu

HEALTHY RECIPES

53 APPETIZERS, SOUPS & SALADS

87 BEEF, PORK & LAMB

123 POULTRY

145 FISH & SEAFOOD

167 EGGS & CHEESE

181 VEGETABLES

197 GRAINS, PASTAS, BEANS & BREADS

219 DESSERTS

248 SPICES

251 INDEX

FORWARD

Ann Hunter, PhD, RD, LD, FADA
Wichita State University

Now that you've invested in a set of Health Craft cookware, it's time to reap the many rewards of hassle-free cooking, delicious meals, and improved health. I know through my years of experience in the food service industry that nothing detracts more from a pleasurable cooking experience than not having the right food to prepare or the right equipment to work with.

As a dietitian, I want my finished entrees to appeal to the eye and the palate, and to meet my clients' nutritional needs. Overcooked vegetables that have lost their color and flavor have little to no nutritional value. Dried out meats that have lost their flavor, are difficult to chew and swallow. With the Health Craft Nutritional Cooking System, you can rest assured that these cooking nightmares won't happen to you. Waterless/Greaseless Cookware retains the valuable vitamins and minerals as well as the natural moisture in your foods.

Because we understand your lifestyle needs, much care went into the selection of the recipes in this cookbook. We recommend you reference the nutritional breakdown of each recipe. For a complete explanation of this breakdown, see page 15. In addition to including the most nutritious entrees, Health Craft has made your variety of choice almost limitless. Choose from a variety of irresistible recipes, such as Singapore Fish, Chicken Satay, Hom Bow, and even Chocolate Mousse.

Part of my role has been determining the nutritional information for each recipe, but through the process I've listed, tasted, and visualized each meal personally. During this project, recipes were improved by reducing fat, sodium, and caloric count, while increasing fiber whenever possible. All this was done without sacrificing the appearance, texture, or taste of the dishes. Each recipe was then retested for taste, quality, and accurate preparation instructions.

So much has been written about nutrition, cholesterol, fats, and diets during the past ten years, it's no wonder we sometimes feel bombarded with information. That's why in this cookbook we've gotten back to the basics of nutrition. You should find the following sections particularly useful: The Surgeon General's report as it relates to foods and nutrition; the Food Guide Pyramid; the basics of metabolism and fats; the new food labels and how to use them; and the calorie point system. We hope you'll turn to these reference pages for years to come.

I've enjoyed my Health Craft cookware for many years and still continue to learn new ways to prepare foods-without added fats and water. You will too! Easily prepared, nutritional meals that are appealing to the eye and the palate... What more could you ask for?

BASIC COOKWARE CARE

Congratulations on your decision to purchase Health Craft "Made in the USA" Nutritional Cooking System. Your decision will pay lifelong dividends in healthful, flavorful and nutritional meals. The vapor seal method of cooking assures you of maximum food value retention, and allows you to prepare your foods without water or added fats. Take a moment now to acquaint yourself with the proper use and care of these fine utensils. By following a few simple steps you will enjoy the maximum benefits and become an expert with the methods of Waterless, Greaseless, Nutritional Cooking.

Cleaning Before First Use

Before using your cookware for the first time, wash each piece thoroughly in warm soapy water with a 1/2 cup of white distilled vinegar added. This initial washing is essential to insure that all manufacturing oils and polishing compounds are removed before cooking food. After this initial washing, normal washing by hand or in a dishwasher is all that is necessary to clean your cookware. Occasional cleaning with a good stainless steel cleaner is recommended.

Daily Care

After each use, wash your cookware in warm soapy water with a dish cloth or nylon plastic net. DO NOT use metal scouring pads, as it may scratch the high polished outside surface or lids of the cookware. If using a metal scouring pad, use it on the inside of the pan only.

Surface Care

Occasionally, when cooking starchy foods or searing meats a stain may appear on the inside surface of the pan. A blue or golden brown discoloration may also appear on the outside of the pan from overheating the unit. These stains are easily removed with a good non-abrasive stainless steel cleaner like Bar Keeper's Friend or Kleen King. First, make a paste with the cleaner and very little water. Then using a paper towel or cloth rub the paste over the stained area, rinse and dry.

During the first few times of use, bright metal marks may appear on the inside of your pans. Remove these and other minor scratches by placing a small amount of Stainless Steel Cleaner into a dry pan, and polish in a circular motion with a damp paper towel or dishcloth. Then clean in warm soapy water, rinse and dry.

While stainless steel is an extremely durable metal, it is not impervious to corrosion, pitting or spotting. Foods such as mustard, mayonnaise, lemon juice, tomatoes, tomato paste, vinegar, salt, dressings, or condiments may etch stainless steel if allowed to remain in contact with the surface for a long period of time. Strong bleaches can have the same effect.

Pitting may result if un-dissolved salt is allowed to remain on the bottom of the pan. Pitting looks like small white spots, and does not in any way affect the performance or usefulness of your pans, nor are they a defect in the metal or the workmanship. To avoid pitting, salt should only be added to the boiling liquid and stirred until it is completely dissolved.

Burned Foods

When finished cooking, fill the pan with warm water and let it soak while you enjoy your meal. If burned foods are not easily removed by normal washing, fill the pan partially full of water and bring to a boil long enough to loosen the food, then clean with stainless steel cleaner, wash with warm soapy water, and dry.

Dried Fruits

Do not place the cover on the pan when cooking sulfur dried foods or food labeled sulfites added as it may stain the cover. Boil liquid 10 minutes prior to covering when cooking these foods.

THE VAPOR SEAL METHOD

Mother Nature designed foods to give us everything we need, naturally. Food contains abundant flavor, vitamins, minerals, digestive enzymes, and color. However, many cooking methods can rob food of its natural qualities.

Fortunately, the Vapor Seal method of Health Craft waterless, greaseless cookware saves money, work, time, energy, flavor, vitamins, minerals and enzymes. "Waterless, Greaseless" cooking is possible because a vapor seal is created around the lid; and heat is distributed evenly across the bottom and up the sides of the cookware.

This process cooks food in its own natural liquids for nutritious, flavor-filled meals. Food shrinkage is greatly reduced, making waterless, greaseless cooking more economical than ordinary cooking methods. The seal is maintained by using low heat. Health Craft cookware is the most energy efficient cookware on the market, and it will pay for itself.

The vapor seal method retains the nutritional value of your foods by eliminating the following process that drains food of its natural goodness. Peeling fruits and vegetables removes the vitamins and minerals directly beneath the skin. We do not recommend you peel these foods; a good scrub with a vegetable brush and water is all that is necessary.

Boiling sterilizes food, dissolves water soluble minerals, and destroys both the flavor and color. The vapor seal method cooks food completely in its own natural moisture, without added water and without boiling.

High temperature destroys vitamins and minerals and causes food to dehydrate and shrink. For example when you smell a roast cooking in the oven you're really smelling the natural meat juices that have been transformed in to vapor. The high temperature combined with open cooking greatly adds to meat shrinkage. The Vapor Seal Method cooks meats on medium to low heat, retaining the natural juices which tenderize and flavor the meat. This method also retains the natural juices and flavor and decreases meat shrinkage dramatically.

Oxidation of food occurs when cooking without a cover exposing food to the air, and reduces the quality of the food significantly. These qualities are locked into the food when the vapor seal is formed, keeping the aroma and natural goodness in the pan. For example, you will not know if broccoli or cabbage is being cooked until the cover is removed from the pan.

Last but not least, adding fat and oil in food preparation make food seven times harder to digest, and it adds excessive calories. Using the vapor seal method, the natural properties of the food keeps it from sticking to the high quality stainless steel pan. Plus the vapor seal method retains natural flavors without the need to add salt, butter or oil after cooking to restore flavor.

The Vapor Seal Cooking Method is very different from traditional cooking methods because you do not need to add moisture or fats. Everything else you already know about cooking applies, once you know the Vapor Seal Method.

Simple Basic Rules

Always use the correct size pan, one that the food nearly fills. Cooking with a pan too large for the food can destroy vitamins and minerals, dry your foods, and possibly cause the food to burn.

Create a Vapor Seal

Fill a pan with fresh or frozen vegetables. Rinse in cold water and drain, the water that clings to the food combine with natural juices to cook the waterless way. Cover the pan, close the vent, and place the pan over low heat. When the cover is hot to the touch and the cover spins freely on a cushion of water, the vapor seal is formed. Continue cooking until done. This is the waterless part of this new cooking method. If you cook several vegetables together with no water there will be no interchange of flavor. Each vegetable will be full of its own flavor and valuable nutrients.

> *TIP: If the heat is too low, the cover will not spin. If the heat is too high, the cover will spit moisture. The vapor seal retains the moisture in your foods with a water seal around the inset cover of the pan. Sometimes when a pan is allowed to cool, the condensed moisture inside the pan creates a vacuum causing the lid to lock onto the pan. Should this happen, simply open the vent.*

Control the Heat

Waterless, greaseless cooking is a lower-temperature method that can be used on any type of range, including the new Induction Cook Tops. Lower heat retains moisture and keeps food from burning. The following are general rules for heat use.

MEDIUM-HIGH HEAT
- For heating utensils to sear or brown meat
- For re-moisturizing dried foods by steaming over water until the water boils.
- For pan broiling thick steaks or chops (½" or thicker)

MEDIUM HEAT
- For pan broiling thin steaks, chops, hamburger or chicken breast
- For quick starting fresh fruits and vegetables until the vapor seal forms
- To start direct top-of-the-range baking

LOW OR SIMMER
- For cooking roasts and meatloaf after browning
- For cooking fresh vegetables and fruits after the vapor seal forms
- For cooking less tender cuts of meat after browning all sides
- For finishing top-of-the-range baking after the pan cover is hot

Don't Peek

Resist the urge to peek: When the cover is removed during the cooking period, heat and moisture escape and the vapor seal is broken. This lengthens the cooking time.

Be Specific

Follow time charts, recipes and general instructions for meats, vegetables, fruits, grains, pasta, desserts, etc., under their specific headings.

Cooking with Gas

Some gas and commercial gas ranges may not allow you to lower the heat enough before the flame goes out. Health Craft is designed to cook at lower temperatures, and cooking at high temperatures may cause your handles to get extremely hot and may even blister. This can be easily solved with a heat diffuser, which defuses the flame, allowing you to cook at lower temperatures.

Cooking Meats without Grease

Begin with meat that is near room temperature. Pre-heat the pan on medium heat for 3-5 minutes. The pan is ready when you can sprinkle a few drops of water in the pan and the water "dances." If the water just evaporates, the pan is not hot enough. Once the pan is hot, place the meat in the pan, pressing against the bottom of the pan, the meat will stick at first. After a short time, it will sear and then loosen from the pan. Turn and sear on the other side. If the meat is not done, or if it is a roast, cover the pan and reduce the heat to low until cooked.

> *TIP: Always roast meat in the smallest utensil into which it will fit. This will result in a tender, juicy cut, and it will shrink less, providing more servings per pound, and savings on food dollars.*

Proper Temperature for Roasting: To obtain the proper cooking temperature for roasting, the cover must spin freely on a cushion of moisture emitting tiny bubbles. If the cover spits moisture, the temperature is too hot.

Top-of-the-Range Baking

Health Craft waterless greaseless cookware is designed to bake cakes, cornbreads, cookies, casseroles, meatloaf, ribs and lasagna in the pan on top of the range more efficiently than in the oven. For example, to bake a small cake, coat the inside of a small fry pan or 2-qt with non-stick cooking spray. Then pour the cake batter into the pan until the pan is half full, cover and close the vent. Set the pan on a burner and adjust the heat to medium. When the lid is hot to touch (about 5 minutes), reduce the heat to low and finish baking (about 10-12 minutes). NOTE: Higher altitudes require longer baking times.

Eggs & Omelets

Some food items with an egg base; fried or scrambled eggs, omelets, pancakes, crepes, French toast, etc., have no natural oil lubricant and will require oil or butter to cook with to prevent sticking. For detailed instruction, see section of Eggs & Cheese.

Stack Cooking

All Health Craft pans are designed to work together. Stack Cooking is one of the ways they do. It is an exciting and very efficient benefit of Health Craft cookware. And it's something you simply cannot do with most other cookware.

Stack Cooking may not be something you do every day, but around the holidays when you have six pans and four burners you'll appreciate this unique feature of your new Health Craft cookware.

Stack Cooking lets you prepare more foods at one time by stacking small pans on top of larger pans on one burner. This is possible because of Health Craft's exceptional heat conductivity, which transfers heat across the bottom and up the sides of your cookware. The high dome Dutch oven cover is made of the same multi-ply full-body material making the perfect surface for stack cooking. Additionally, your gourmet Chef Pans invert to form high dome Dutch oven covers on a number of the saucepans, stockpots and skillets. Only Health Craft cookware has this feature.

Here's an example of Stack Cooking:
- Begin cooking a roast as normal in the 6-quart or 8-quart Stockpot; sear it on all sides then place accompanying vegetables around it.
- Lower the heat and set the Steamer Rack in the Stockpot. Put a prepared cake mix in the Double-Boiler or Cake Pan and place it on the Steamer Rack. Cover with the high dome Dutch oven cover.
- Pre-heat a small saucepan of frozen vegetables or cored apples on medium heat, cover and close the vent. When the lid is hot to the touch, turn off the burner under the small saucepan and set it on top of the high dome Dutch oven cover to continue cooking.

This entire meal will cook in about 50 minutes — on one burner.

BASIC PRODUCT INFORMATION

Health Craft waterless, greaseless cookware, in many ways, is different from both the less expensive pots and pans on display in discount stores and the popular commercially designed cookware available in the upscale market. First and foremost, waterless, greaseless cookware is designed for the home cook. Secondly, it's not available in retail stores. Historically it has only been available through Cooking Show Hosts who either come to your home for a private cooking lesson, or through healthy cooking demonstrations at Consumer Tradeshows. Why this method of marketing? Prior to our series of cookbooks, there was no other way besides a live cooking demonstration to explain the values and principles of waterless, greaseless cooking. Today, waterless, greaseless cookware is available on the internet. Beware, not all of the cookware that claims to be waterless and greaseless is truly waterless and greaseless.

The quality and workmanship of waterless, greaseless cookware varies from company to company and from set to set, as do the features and benefits. We know firsthand that good cookware is expensive to manufacture, and as the designer and manufacturer of America's premier line of waterless, greaseless cookware "Health Craft", there is no such thing as getting more than what you pay for. Authentic waterless, greaseless cookware is expensive but no more so than the popular commercially designed cookware, and certainly equal to the value of the refrigerator you use to keep your foods fresh and the range you use to cook with. Health Craft waterless, greaseless cookware is more than a lifetime investment: it's an investment in a healthy lifestyle.

When purchasing waterless, greaseless cookware, purchase from a reputable company and a reputable individual. You can always tell a company by the people it keeps and by how long they've been with the company. And even more important, compare features, facts and benefits before you buy. Believe it or not, American manufacturers still make the best cookware on the market today.

Features to Consider

Waterless, greaseless cookware is available in many styles, brand names, and price points. The best performing are the induction compatible surgical stainless steel with Multi-Ply Full Body aluminum core, and weighted vented covers that form the essential *Vapor Seal* for waterless cooking.

Surgical stainless steel alloys combine chromium, nickel, vanadium, titanium and steel to create a hard outer ply surface that is durable, resistant to wear, easy to clean, sanitary, and can be highly polished for an attractive, permanent finish.

Multi-ply full body aluminum core Health Craft pans are excellent heat conductors, providing the most efficient use of energy while cooking. They spread heat evenly to prevent hot spots, and the surgical stainless steel cooking surface keep food from sticking and burning.

Beyond the vapor seal advantage, waterless, greaseless cookware should be designed with every concern of the modern kitchen user in mind. Once you own a good set of waterless, greaseless cookware, it will be very difficult to settle for less.

Here's what to look for:

Full-Body Construction, the pans should be the same Multi-Ply material across the bottom and up the sides of pan, to the rim.

Induction Compatible 'Green Cookware', even though you may not be familiar with Induction Cook Tops, more than likely you WILL have one in your home within the next five to ten years, so it's important to select cookware that is induction compatible. Induction cook tops work using a magnetic principle that heats the pan, not the cook top, and are 80% more energy efficient than gas or electric.

When selecting a brand, *self storing covers,* where the lids can be inverted and **nest perfectly** inside the rim of the pan for easy storage should be a consideration.

The pan should have a **Vapor Vent** for cooking chicken, steaks and chops to a golden brown with the cover on and the vent open, preventing grease splatter. Vegetables will cook in their own juices to save vitamins and minerals forming a vapor seal with the vent closed.

Burn Safe Knobs and Finger Guards, the top knob should rest on a finger guard to prevent your fingers from touching the hot lid. Both the knob and the finger guard should be made of heat resistant material that will handle oven temperatures up to 350°F (on bake). The top knob insert should also have a stainless steel or brass fitting to prevent stripping. The handles and top knobs should be dishwasher safe. Metal handles should be made of a non-magnetic stainless steel to prevent the handle from heating to the same temperature of the pan when used on an Induction Range.

Handle Fitting should be protected by a stainless steel flame guard between the handle and pan. Attachment by stainless steel fittings welded to the pan will ensure stability, resistant to corrosion, stay tight and locked into position. Health Craft features both a push-button and spring loaded handles that can be easily removed, turning the pans into Bakeware. No screws to loosen.

Self Serving Covers where the cover lid can be inverted so the pan will balance on the lid as a trivet, **for Informal Dining.**

Rivets and Rolled Edges - No rivets should penetrate the inside of the pans. Bacteria from grease and food particles can become trapped around rivets, making such a pan design much more difficult to clean. Rolled edges around the top of the rim also trap food, grease and bacteria. Edges should be smooth and polished for easy cleaning and sanitation.

Warp resistant Bottoms - The bottom of the pans should be designed to assure the utensil hugs the burner for maximum heat efficiency, but should also be slightly concave (paneled) in the center so the pan will flatten out when heated and contract when cooled to prevent warping, making the pans practical for use on all types of ranges, including smooth glass top surfaces and the new induction cook-tops.

Product Warranty – Cookware designs and styles come and go so do cookware companies. When selecting a new set or collection of waterless cookware it's important to know how long the company has been in business. The best way to determine this is by research and asking 'How long' the rep has been with the company.

Induction Cooking

Health Craft uses the principles of electromagnetism to heat the T430 magnetic Surgical Stainless Steel on the outside, transferring heat quickly and efficiently to the inside. Induction Technology offers levels of efficiency, control and safety unavailable from electric and gas cook-tops or microwave ovens. With ever increasing energy costs Induction Cookware is quickly becoming the choice of millions of homeowners and professionals worldwide.

The induction cook-top has inductor coils under the ceramic surface, when a pan is set on the range an electric current passes through the coil creating a pulsing magnetic field. The metals of the pan have a natural resistance to the movement of electrons causing the pan to heat up.

It's the pan, not the cook-top that heats up and cooks the food. Nothing outside the pan is affected by the magnetic field. As soon as the pan is removed, the range shuts off, and heat generation ceases immediately.

If you donot have an Induction Cooktop at this writing, more than likely you will within the next five to ten years. When purchasing waterless, greaseless cookware, be sure it's Induction Compatible. The best test is to place a magnet on the side of the pan.

Seven (7) key advantages of Health Craft Induction Cookware:

FASTER because energy is directly transferred within the pan's T430 Surgical Stainless Steel metal, heating is faster than gas!

SAFER because there is no open flame, red-hot coil or other radiant heat source to ignite fumes or flammable materials, Health Craft Cookware helps to prevent burns and kitchen fires.

CLEANER because with no grates or carbon build-up to worry about, clean up is a breeze; just use a damp cloth and wipe over the smooth, easy-to-clean ceramic glass surface.

COOLER because gas ranges produce unused heat that goes into your kitchen, increasing your cooling costs, with Health Craft Induction Cookware, almost no wasted heat is produced since all the heat is being generated within the pan itself.

CHEAPER because 80% of every dollar you spend on energy goes right into the pan! Gas delivers 43% of the energy you pay for to the pan and electric about 44 to 53%. Plus, when you remove the pan from the induction surface, the unit immediately goes into standby mode, using virtually no energy whatsoever.

EVEN HEATING because the T430 magnetic stainless steel on the outside of the Health Craft cookware heats at the same level uniformly, there can be no hot spots. The computerized monitoring feature allows maximum heating of the pan.

PORTABLE the Health Craft Induction Cooking Unit can be used safely and efficiently anywhere, including a boat or recreational vehicle.

BASIC U.S./METRIC CONVERSIONS

The recipes in this cookbook are U.S. standard measurements. Appropriate metric equivalents are also provided with each recipe. For small quantities, customary tablespoon and teaspoon measurements are used in the recipes.

For easy reference, the following metric conversions have been rounded to provide convenient working measurements.

Weight

U.S.		Metric
1 ounce		30 grams
4 ounces		115 grams
8 ounces		230 grams
16 ounces	(1 pound)	460 grams
32 ounces	(2 pounds)	1 kilogram

Oven Temperature

U.S.	Metric
200°F	90°C
225°F	110°C
250°F	120°C
275°F	135°C
300°F	150°C
350°F	180°C
375°F	190°C
400°F	210°C

Volume Measurements

U.S.		Metric
teaspoon to milliliter		
1/4 tsp		1.5 ml
1/2 tsp		3 ml
1 tsp		5 ml
1 1/2 tsp		7.5 ml
2 tsp		10 ml
2 1/2 tsp		12.5 ml
tablespoon to milliliter		
1 tbls		15 ml
1 1/2 tbls		22.5 ml
2 tbls		30 ml
cup to milliliter		
1/4 cup		60 ml
1/3 cup		80 ml
1/2 cup		120 ml
2/3 cup		160 ml
3/4 cup		180 ml
1 cup		240 ml
4 cups	(1 quart)	1 liter

Imperial/Australian Equivalents

Other		Metric
1	Imperial 1/2 pint (10 oz)	300 ml
1	Australian cup (8 oz)	240 ml
Note:	*1.25 U.S. cup 10 oz =*	
	1 Imperial 1/2 pint	

RECIPE FEATURES

Each recipe found in all of our cookbooks and website provides quick, at-a-glance nutritional information, in the same place on every recipe page. This feature allows you to quickly see all the information you need. For instance, preparation time is the second feature for every recipe. If you have a surprise guests for dinner, or an unexpected interruption – this feature lets you know quickly if you have enough time to prepare the recipe.

Number of Servings: If the recipe is designed for eight servings and you know you need only four, divide all the ingredients in half before preparing.

Equipment: The proper cooking utensil is called for in every recipe. Never again will you be pouring from one pan to another because there is not enough room in the first utensil.

> *NOTE: On the side of every Health Craft pan, under the logo, you will find the name or the designation of that particular pan. No other cookware provides that information.*

Ingredients: everything you need is in one column – no searching necessary. Additionally all ingredients are listed for U.S. and metric measures when appropriate, making converting unnecessary.

Preparation: Short, to-the-point descriptions of each step.

Nutritional Breakdowns: Anyway you measure your nutritional needs – by calories, by grams, by percent of total or the calorie point system – it can be found always in the same order, always in the same place.

Example of Breakdowns:

> **NUTRITIONAL BREAKDOWN PER SERVING:** Calories 292; Fat Grams 7; Carbohydrate Grams 45; Protein Grams 13; Cholesterol mg 69; Sodium mg 140.

> **THE POINT SYSTEM:** Calorie Points 4; Protein Points 2; Fat Grams 7; Sodium Points 6; Fiber Points 1; Carbohydrate Points 3; Cholesterol Points 7.

NOTE: Method used for nutritional information was Nutritionist IV software, N-Square Computing and Food Values of Portions Commonly Used by Jean A. T. Pennington.

ADAPTING RECIPES

Many cooks put a lot of pressure on themselves when it comes to preparing a meal. They must have a recipe to follow and it must be followed to the tee. Although the stores and internet are full of cookbooks, only Health Craft publishes detailed cookbooks, instructions and recipes on waterless, greaseless cooking, and all of our cookbooks are written by professionals.

To enjoy the recipes and receive the benefits of cooking without water and added fats, you will need to learn to adapt recipes. The easiest way to do this is to understand and trust your Health Craft cookware.

Use Lower Temperature Settings

One of the benefits of Health Craft waterless, greaseless, induction cookware, with full-body construction, is the way it conducts heat – on low. One common mistake is using a heat setting that is too high. Keep this in mind – a perfect cake can bake on top of the range on LOW about 200°F. To bake the same cake in the oven would require 350°F (180°C)! The full body construction of Health Craft multi-core waterless, greaseless, induction cookware goes across the bottom and up the sides of the pan, to the rim, conducting heat evenly, requiring low temperatures. Think of a full-body constructed pan and cover a as a mini-oven on top of the stove. Leave the cover in place, the same as you leave an oven door shut, and close the vent. To bake cakes, spray the pan with non-stick cooking spray (or lightly oil) – fill the pan half full with batter, and cover (vent closed). Start cooking on medium heat for five minutes then reduce heat to low, and cook according to half the time listed on recipe directions. The average time to bake a cake in Health Craft cookware is about 15 - 20 minutes.

Understanding Waterless Cooking

Rinse and freshen vegetables. Pour off excess water, cover utensil, close vent, set on low heat, and remember not to peek. Every time you lift the cover you allow the moisture to escape. Be sure you are using the correct size pan. The vegetables should fill or almost fill the pan. When too much air is inside the pan, the vapor seal will not form, and the vegetables may burn.

If the food has its own moisture, like vegetables and fruits, you can retain the moisture cooking with low heat, the cover on and the vent closed. If the food is dried, such as rice, pasta, or dried beans; you will need to add liquid to rehydrate.

Some Recipes Need Water

There are always a few... One afternoon our customer service department received a frantic phone call. *"My Pasta is burning and smoking!"* Some recipes require water or liquid; beans, rice, pasta and naturally soup, stews and sauces. Remember, Waterless for vegetables and greaseless for meat, poultry, and some seafood.

Enjoy Greaseless Cooking

You may prepare your foods WITHOUT added oils and fats. Remember, you are cooking on a surgical stainless steel surface. To prepare steaks, chops and poultry; preheat the utensil on medium to medium-high heat until water drops "dance" when sprinkled in the pan. Place meat in the pan (take care in positioning, as the meat will immediately begin to sear, temporarily sticking to the hot surface). After 4 or 5 minutes try to lift the corner of the meat, do not force it, the meat will release when that side is seared. Turn and sear to your preference.

To sauté onions and garlic, simply use low heat, cover the pan, and close the vent – they sauté in their own moisture... no oil is needed. If olive oil is added, it's added for the flavor so often less is used. Most meats, poultry, chops, and fish have natural fats and oils, so you do not need to add it. Eggs have no natural oil – you need to spray the pan with cooking spray or use a small amount of unsalted butter or margarine.

Practice Regular Cleaning

Use a stainless steel cleaner regularly. Your Health Craft cookware performs best, and food will not stick, when cleaned properly. Barkeeper's Friend is available in most stores and Health Craft stainless steel cleaner can be purchased online at www.healthcraft.com "Shop online".

Roasting on top of the Stove

Cooking time is for unstuffed, skinned poultry, as well as beef, pork and lamb, is reduced by about half the time. Begin with meat that is nearly room temperature. To roast, preheat appropriate size utensil over medium or medium-high heat (depending on range type). Sear first side of meat, covered with vent open. After the first side is seared (caramelized) turn meat when it releases easily from the pan, reduce heat to low. With the high dome in place (or cover with vent closed), roast to desired doneness using the methods described on the previous page. Proper roasting temperature can be determined by tiny bubbles forming around the base of the cover. If water bubbles spit, reduce the temperature so only tiny bubbles appear around the rim. Cooking time begins after searing (browning) the meat on all sides and covering.

Minutes per lb.	Desired doneness	Internal Temperature*
8	Rare	
9	Medium Rare	145°F (65°C)
10	Medium	165°F (70°C)
11	Medium-Well	
12	Well-Done	170°F (75°C)

*Internal cooking temperatures established by USDA

Pan Broiling Chicken, Steaks and Chops

To cook meats and some fish the greaseless way: Preheat appropriate size skillet over medium-high heat until water droplets "dance" on the pan. Place meats in the pan lightly pressing down to ensure meat surface is in contact with the surface of the pan. Cover the pan and open the vent. Meat will immediately begin to sear, initially sticking to the pan. When first side is seared (3-5 minutes) meats will loosen, turn over and sear other side for additional 3-5 minutes. **Test for Doneness.**

To deglaze for creating a *pan sauce*; after removing meats add 1 cup (80 ml) of liquid (chicken stock, beef stock, veal stock or wine) and stir to loosen juices from pan. Pour over meats. For a thicker sauce, reduce over medium-high heat until desired thickness.

Testing Meat for Doneness

During the searing and Pan Broiling of steaks, chops, and poultry, when you cook with the cover on and the vent open; the meat will cook quicker and juicier. However, crowding the pan, or cooking at too low a temperature and covering, may cause the meat to steam. Practice makes perfect, and a good home cook quickly learns to cook steaks, chops and poultry to the desired doneness with good equipment, proper techniques, and by feel. Because of the different texture, cuts and thickness, learning the feel of the desired doneness by pushing down on the center of the cut of meat with a fork is by far the best method over attempting to time for doneness, or cutting into the meat and releasing the natural juices. These basic rules apply to cooking all meats when attempting to accomplish different stages of doneness. To demonstrate, turn the palm of your left hand up and spread your fingers apart.

Doneness Tests

Rare: Rest your left thumb against your left forefinger and press down on the soft fleshy part at the base of your left thumb with your right forefinger. That's what <u>rare</u> feels like.

Medium-Rare: Place your left thumb directly over the center of your left forefinger and press down on the soft fleshy part at the base of your left thumb with your right forefinger. That's what <u>medium-rare</u> feels like.

Medium: Place your left thumb in between your left forefinger and your left middle finger and press down on the soft fleshy part at the base of your left thumb with your right forefinger. That's what <u>medium</u> feels like.

<u>Medium-Well:</u> Place your left thumb directly over the center of your left middle finger and press down on the soft fleshy part at the base of your left thumb with your right forefinger. That's what medium-well feels like.

Pan Frying Seafood and floured and breaded Meats

Pan frying with a small amount of oil or unsalted butter is recommended for floured and breaded meats, as well as most seafood. With the exception of Tuna, Salmon and Sword Fish, (which can be pan broiled the greaseless way in a similar method to steaks, chops and chicken), most seafood contains very little natural oils. Add a little oil or butter prior to adding seafood, floured or breaded meats to the pan. Fry over medium to medium-high heat. Cook about 3-5 minutes per side, and Test for desired Doneness.

Steaming and Braising Meats

There are a few exceptions to cooking meats the waterless and greaseless way. Some recipes call for braising or steaming meats. Steaming can be an excellent method to remove excess fat from ground beef, lamb or venison. Live lobster, crab, mussels, and clams are also best cooked by steaming or braising (submerging in liquid).

> **To Steam Meats:** Place the 6-quart Steamer/Pasta Basket in the 'tall' 6½-quart Stockpot, add 2-3 cups of water, stock, wine or beer, and bring to a boil over medium-high heat. Add meat to Steamer/Pasta basket and cover with the vent open, about 15 minutes per pound. Live Lobster, Crabs, Mussels and Clams are best steamed in wine or beer. When the alcohol is released during the boiling process the seafood is gently put to sleep, relaxing the muscles and tenderizing the meat, then cooked to perfection.

Braising is the process of submerging the meat in stocks, wine, beer or water.

Fruits and Vegetables the Waterless Way

No Need to Peel... With Health Craft waterless, greaseless cooking, delicious fruits and vegetables can be prepared without sacrificing the wonders of nature. The first major breakthrough of this unique cooking method eliminates the need to strip away the flavor-and nutrient-rich skin. For most fruits and vegetables, a gentle scrub is all that's needed before cooking. One more step to ensure that all of nature's goodness arrive garden fresh at your table.

Lower Heat

The second major breakthrough of the Health Craft waterless, greaseless method eliminates the devastating damage caused by high-heat oil sautéing, boiling, or microwaving of vegetables. High heat destroys most of the health-giving water-and fat-soluble minerals along with the very delicate flavors and colors, not to mention the life giving enzymes. The vegetable's most valuable nutritional advantages are often thrown out with the cooking oil or water.

With Health Craft waterless, greaseless "flavor-sealing" covered utensils and heavy-duty construction; vegetables can be cooked with low heat, eliminating the need for boiling in water and sautéing in oil. With low heat, the vegetables are cooked "waterless" quickly and evenly in a vacuum below the boiling temperature, or "greaseless" without oil, and prepared in their own natural moisture. Using the vegetable's natural juices eliminates the need to add water or oil during cooking.

Less Oxidation

The third major breakthrough of Health Craft waterless cooking is the elimination of harmful oxidation. Detrimental oxidation occurs when vegetables are boiled or steamed in uncovered utensils, pressure-cooked or cooked in a microwave, allowing a good share of the health-giving properties to evaporate.

21

The waterless feature of Health Craft, with its unique vapor-sealing covers, locks vitamins, minerals and enzymes in the utensil. No steam is allowed to escape. Wonderful aromas remain inside the pan. Until the cover is removed, you won't know if its broccoli or cabbage being prepared. The vegetables cook on low heat, cooking evenly in their own natural moisture, below the boiling temperature.

Scrub Root Vegetables
To clean root vegetables, scrub vigorously with a vegetable brush under cold running water and remove any surface blemishes with a paring knife. Do not peel.

Refresh Vegetables
All fresh vegetables, especially root vegetables, have a tendency to lose some of their natural moisture after harvesting. To add back some of the lost moisture, place the vegetables in the pan, fill the pan with water, add 1 tablespoon of white distilled vinegar and soak for 10 to 15 minutes. Soaking also removes chemical sprays, preservatives and any other substance the vegetable may have come in contact with in transit and in storage. Pour the water off, rinse and cook according to the recipe.

Use the Right-Size Pan
When cooking vegetables the waterless way, it's very important to use a pan that the vegetables nearly fill. This is an essential step in forming the vapor seal. When there are fewer vegetables in the pan, the more air, which can cause oxidation, and less-full pans will require higher temperature settings to create a vapor seal, and more than likely, the vegetables will be scorched or burned.

Form the Vapor Seal
As the moist air inside the pan is heated, it expands and is forced out between the rim and the cover of the pan. Around the rim is a well, or reservoir, that collects moisture. The covers are angled down to fit perfectly in line with the well. As the heated air continues to escaped, the well is filled with moisture, forming the vapor seal. This usually takes 3 to 5 minutes.

Find the Right Temperature Setting
Whether you have an electric range with a glass top, European or conventional burners, or a conventional or commercial gas range, or the new induction range, Health Craft cookware takes all the guesswork out of cooking the waterless way.

Here are some tips, "with the Vapor Vent Closed":
  If the rim or well spits moisture, the temperature is too high.
  If the lid does not spin freely on a cushion of water after forming the vapor seal, the temperature is too low.

Once you discover the proper setting for your range, cooking the waterless way will be simple and easy. If you have a commercial gas range and you cannot achieve sufficient low temperatures for cooking vegetables the waterless, greaseless way, use a Trivet or "Flame Tamer" placed over your burner. You can also call your dealer and ask that they replace your commercial gas burners with those specifically and safely designed for the home kitchen.

Don't Peek

During the waterless cooking process, don't peek. Removing the cover will destroy the vapor seal; lengthen the cooking time and may cause the vegetables to burn. If you or another member of the family does lift the lid, cover the pan, close the vent and add 2 tablespoons water to the rim to reestablish the vapor seal. Add 3 to 5 minutes to the prescribed cooking time. Most important, trust your new Health Craft cookware.

Cooking Fresh Vegetables the Waterless Way

To cook, place the vegetables in a pan that they nearly fill. Rinse with cold water and pour the water off. The water that clings to the vegetables and its own natural moisture are sufficient for cooking the waterless way.

Cover the pan, close the vent and cook over medium-low heat. When the cover spins freely on a cushion of water, the vapor seal has formed. Cook according to the time chart. Don't peak. Removing the cover will destroy the vapor seal; lengthen the cooking time and may cause the vegetables to burn. If at first you are concerned about cooking without water, add 2 or 3 tablespoons of water to the pan after rinsing and cook as directed. As your confidence builds, you can lessen the amount of water used.

When finished cooking, test for doneness with a fork. If not done, cover the pan, close the vent and add 2 tablespoons of water to the rim to reestablish the vapor seal. Cook over low heat for 5 to 10 minutes.

Cooking Frozen Vegetables the Waterless Way!

Do not defrost. Place the frozen vegetables in the pan they most nearly fill. Rinse with cold water and pour the water off. The water that clings to the vegetables and its own natural moisture are sufficient for cooking the waterless way.

Cover the pan, close the vent and cook over medium-low heat. When the cover spins freely on a cushion of water, the vapor seal has formed. Cook according to the time chart. Don't peak. Removing the cover will destroy the vapor seal; lengthen the cooking time and may cause the vegetables to burn.

Cooking for One or Two

When cooking for one or two people, naturally the quantity of vegetables will be less. However, with waterless cooking more than one vegetable can be cooked in the same pan with no interchanging of flavors or colors. You can cook potatoes, sliced carrots and broccoli all in the same pan the waterless way. For example, using a 1 or 1 ¼-quart covered saucepan, place the potatoes in the pan, halved or whole, with the skin side to the surface of the pan, add two carrots (sliced) and top with frozen corn and broccoli florets. Rinse the vegetables and pour the water off. Cook as directed above.

Cooking Times for Fresh Vegetables

Scrub root vegetables and remove blemishes. Do not peel; peeling removes valuable minerals and vitamins. Place vegetables in pan they most nearly fill.

Vegetable	Cooking Time*
Artichokes	30-45 minutes
Asparagus	10-15 minutes
Beans, Yellow & Green	20-25 minutes
Beans, Lima	30-35 minutes
Beets, whole	35-40 minutes
Broccoli	15-20 minutes
Brussel Sprouts	15-20 minutes
Cabbage, shredded	10-15 minutes
Carrots, sliced	15-20 minutes
Cauliflower	10-15 minutes
Chinese Pea Pods	3-5 minutes
Corn**	10-12 minutes
Eggplant	5-8 minutes
Greens	10-12 minutes
Leeks	12-15 minutes
Mushrooms	4-5 minutes
Okra	15-20 minutes
Onions, whole	15-20 minutes
Parsnips, sliced	15-20 minutes
Peas	5-7 minutes
Potatoes, White, quartered*	20-25 minutes
Potatoes, Sweet*	30-35 minutes

Potatoes, baked*	30-35 minutes
Spinach	8-10 minutes
Squash, summer	15-20 minutes
Squash, winter	25-30 minutes
Tomatoes	10-15 minutes
Turnips, Rutabagas	25-30 minutes

Potatoes, sweet potatoes and yams can be cut into halves or quarters to shorten cooking time, place skin side against the utensil. To avoid scorching, place a paper towel on the bottom of the pan. Fill the pan with potatoes, rinse and pour off the excess moisture. Cover, close the vent and cook over medium-low heat until the vapor seal is formed (approximately 3-5 minutes). Continue cooking according to the chart below. Cooking time begins when vapor seal is formed.

**For corn on the cob, remove husks and silks, Cover the bottom of the utensil with husks. Place corn in layers on husks, rinse and pour water off, cover, close the vent, and form vapor seal over low heat. To keep your vegetables hot and ready to serve, keep the cover on and the vent closed. The vegetables will stay hot in the pan for 30 minutes or more.

How to Cook Perfect Pasta

An exception to the rule of waterless cooking, pasta must be cooked in rapidly boiling water so that individual pieces can float freely; otherwise they will stick together and cook unevenly. Using the 6 ½-quart "Tall" Stockpot and 6-quart Pasta/Steamer Basket, allow 4 quarts of water for 1 pound of pasta. Never try to boil more than 1½ pounds at a time. It will not cook or drain properly.

Oil added to the water does not prevent pasta from sticking together, it only coats the pasta, preventing it from fully absorbing the water, and the sauce after draining.

When draining pasta, reserve at least half a cup of the cooking water. The pasta will continue to absorb moisture after draining, and it may be necessary to add some of the cooking water to the serving bowl so that sauce and pasta combine well.

Fresh Pasta

For 1 pound (500g) of pasta: Bring 4 quarts of water to a boil. Add 1 teaspoon salt, and the pasta. Stir the pasta and then cover the pan, open the vent. Bring back to a boil, cook for 5 seconds for fine noodles, 15 seconds for thicker cuts. Total cooking time should not exceed 2 minutes, or 3~5 minutes for stuffed pasta. Drain the pasta without delay. Combine the pasta with the sauce, adding some of the reserved cooking water, if necessary.

Dried Pasta

Cooking dried pasta in too little water crowds the pan as the pasta swells, making it stick together. For 1 pound (500g) of pasta: Bring 4 quarts of water to a boil in the 6 1/5-quart "Tall" Stockpot with 6-quart Pasta/Steamer Basket inserted. Add 1 teaspoon salt (under-salted or unsalted pasta is virtually tasteless). Cook according to the times printed on the package, lift a piece out and taste to see if al dente (firm to the bite).

Whole Grain Pasta

Cooking enriched grain and whole grain dried pasta may require 2 to 5 minutes additional cooking time respectively, and should be cooked al dente.

Pasta Dictionary

Acini di pepe: "Peppercorns"; tiny little solid beads.

Anellini: "Little Rings"

Bows: The American version of Italian farfalle, or "Butterflies"; often egg noodle dough.

Cannelloni: Large cylinders stuffed with a variety of fillings.

Capellini: Means "fine hairs," very delicate round noodles; sometimes called capelli d'angelo, or "angel hair." Capellini Tagliati: Broken angel hair.

Cavatelli: A short curled noodle, available fresh, frozen, and dried; the dried are shell shaped with a slightly ruffled outside.

Conchiglie: See description for 'Shells'.

Conchigliette: Little Shells; for soups with vegetables or lentils.

Couscous: Granules of pasta made from semolina flour. Couscous is typically cooked by steaming over boiling water or used in a stew.

Coralli: Tiny tubes, similar to Tubettini.

Ditaloni Rigati: "Little thimbles" ridged or smooth, used in soups with beans.

Egg Noodles: Ribbons in varying widths.

Elbow Macaroni: Narrow, curved tubes, about 1 inch.

Farfalle/Butterflies: See description for 'Bows.'

Fedelini: Very fine ribbon pasta, similar to vermicelli.

Fettuccini: Long, flat, ribbon-shaped, about $\frac{1}{8}$-inch wide.

Fusilli: Long, fat, spiral-shaped spaghetti. For meat sauces and baked pasta dishes.

Gamelli: Means "twins," because it looks like two short fat pieces of spaghetti twisted together.

Gnocchi: Dumplings filled with ricotta or mashed potatoes, served with tomato, butter, or meat sauces.

Lasagna: Large, flat noodles about 3-inches wide with curly edges.

Linguine: Thin, slightly flat, solid strands, about $\frac{1}{8}$ – inch wide, for white and red clam sauce, pesto, and oil-based sauces.

Macaroni: Thin, tubular, in various widths; may be long like spaghetti or shorter lengths.

Manicotti: Thick, ridged tubes, cut straight or on an angle.

Messani: A tubular pasta 1 to 2 inches (2.5 to 5 cm) long with a smooth exterior; the same pasta with ridged exterior is call Mezzani Rigati.

Mostaccioli: Means "small mustaches," cut looks like penne.

Orecchiette: "Little ears," round and fat, for thick, rustic sauces or with vegetable sauces and ragu.

Orzo: Tiny pasta shape that resembles large grains of rice.

Pastina: Very tiny grains of dough; for soup.

Penne Grandi (Sardi): Large tube shapes are for use with ragu, meat, and robust vegetable sauces containing broccoli or cauliflower.

Penne Lisce: For chunky tomato sauces, meat sauces, and cream sauces.

Penne Mezzanine: The smallest penne, for light vegetable sauces and tomato sauces.

Penne Rigate: Ridged, for butter based sauces, meat or vegetable creations, and cheese sauces.

Perciatelli: A fatter version of Bucatini.

Quadretinni: Small flat squares.

Ramen noodles: used extensively in Japan, although Chinese in origin. For Japanese noodle soups. The fresh noodles need to be boiled until they are tender before adding to soup. Dried instant noodles only need boiling water poured over them to be cooked.

Rice Noodles: Various widths (up to about $\frac{1}{8}$ inch), long, straight ribbons, and rice vermicelli, very thin.

Riso: Orzo, rosamarina

Ravioli: Stuffed squares of pasta filled; cheese, vegetable, or meat fillings, usually made by hand, or bought fresh.

Rigatoni: Thick- ridged tubes for meat and sausage sauces, fresh tomato sauces, vegetable sauces, and baked timbale.

Rotella: Spiral shaped. Sometime call fusilli.

Rotini: Small, round, 6-spoked wheels for meat and cheese sauces.

Semi di mela; "Apple seed"

Shells: Available from tiny to jumbo; called conchiglie and maruzze.

Spaghetti: Solid, round strands ranging from very thin to thin; for spaghetti sauce, fish sauces, or oil-based sauces.

Spaghettini: Same as spaghetti, but thinner.

Taglierini: Paper-thin, ribbon about 1/16-inch wide; also known as tagliarini, tagliolini, and tonnarelli.

Tortellini: Little pies. Made from 2-inch disks of pasta and filled with either meat or cheese.

Tubettini: Little tubes used in light soups.

Vermicelli: Very fine cylindrical, similar to capellini and fedelini, broken up, for broth-based soups. Thicker varieties are suitable for sauces.

Ziti: Medium-size tubes; for ragu and meat and vegetable sauces, and baking.

Grains

Foods made from grains (wheat, rice, and oats) help form the foundation of a nutritious diet. They provide vitamins, minerals, carbohydrates (starch and dietary fiber), and other substances that are important for good health. Grain products are low in fat, unless fat is added in processing, in preparation, or at the table. Whole grains differ from refined grains in the amount of fiber and nutrients they provide, and different whole grain foods differ in nutrient content, so choose a variety of whole and enriched grains. Eating plenty of whole grains, such as whole wheat bread or oatmeal as part of the healthful eating patterns described by these guidelines, may help protect you against many chronic diseases. Aim for at least 6 servings of grain products per day—more if you are an older child or teenager, an adult man, or an active woman and include several servings of whole grain foods.

Why choose Whole Grain foods?

Vitamins, minerals, fiber, and other protective substances in whole grain foods contribute to the health benefits of whole grains. Refined grains are low in fiber and in the protective substances that accompany fiber. Eating plenty of fiber-containing foods, such as whole grains (and also many fruits and vegetables) promotes proper bowel function. The high fiber content of many whole grains may also help you to feel full with fewer calories. Fiber is best obtained from foods like whole grains, fruits, and vegetables rather than from fiber supplements for several reasons: there are many types of fiber, the composition of fiber is poorly understood, and other protective substances accompany fiber in foods.

Cooking Instructions

Bring liquid to a boil over medium heat, add grain, stir, cover and close vent, reduce the heat to low for required cooking time. Do not stir again. Fluff with a fork to separate grains before serving. Grains are also an excellent choice for Stack Cooking. Bring liquid to a boil over medium heat, add grain, stir, cover and close vent, and stack on top of another pan converted to a Dutch oven.

BASIC COOKING INSTRUCTIONS

Grain	Grain & Liquid	Metric	Cooking Time	Yields
Amaranth	I cup & 3 cups	720 ml	25 minutes	2 ½ cups
Barley, Flaked	I cup & 3 cups	720 ml	15 minutes	3 cups
Barley, Pearled	I cup & 2 ½ cups	600 ml	30-40 minutes	2 ½ cups
Buckwheat Groats	I cup & 2 cups	480 ml	10 minutes	3 ½ cups
Bulgur	I cup & 2 cups	480 ml	15 minutes	2 ½ cups
Cornmeal	I cup & 4 cups	960 ml	30 minutes	3 cups
Couscous	I cup & I ⅔ cups	400 ml	5 minutes*	3 cups
Farina	3 tbls & I cup	240 ml	½ minute	I cup
Millet	I cup & 3 cups	720 ml	20 minutes	4 ½ cups
Oat Groats	I cup & 3 cups	720 ml	40 minutes	2 ½ cups
Oats, Rolled	I cup & 2 cups	480 ml	15 minutes	4 cups
Oats, Quick	I cup & 2 cups	480 ml	1 minute	2 cups
Quinoa	I cup & 2 cups	480 ml	15 minutes	3 ½ cups
Rice, Brown	I cup & 2 cups	480 ml	35 minutes	2 ½ cups
Rice, White	I cup & 2 cups	480 ml	30 minutes	2 ½ cups
Rice, Instant	I cup & I cup	240 ml	5 minutes*	2 cups
Rice, Parboiled	¼ cup & ½ cup	120 ml	20 minutes	I cup
Rice, Wild	I cup & 4 cups	960 ml	50 minutes	3 ½ cups
Rye, Flakes	I cup & 2 cups	480 ml	15 minutes	4 cups
Rye, Berries	I cup & 2 cups	480 ml	60 minutes	2 ½ cups
Soy Grits	I cup & I cup	240 ml	5 minutes*	2 cups
Wheat Berries	I cup & 2 cups	480 ml	60 minutes	2 ½ cups
Wheat, Cracked	I cup & 2 ½ cups	600 ml	30 minutes	3 cups

*Add hot liquid, cover, close the vent, and remove from heat.

Eggs, Omelets and Crepes

This is an exception to greaseless cooking method. Having no natural oils, a small amount of lubricant like unsalted butter, margarine or oil, is required to prevent eggs and egg based recipes from sticking to the pan. Secondly, the pan must be clean, and last but not least, the heat must be adjusted to medium or medium-high heat to cook. We suggest the use of unsalted butter as a lubricant and to achieve the proper cooking temperature for eggs. If the butter burns, the pan is too hot. Once you have learned the proper cooking temperature, you may use oil or margarine as a lubricant.

Frying Eggs

Preheat the 7-inch gourmet Chef Pan over medium heat. Place a small amount of unsalted butter in the pan, enough to cover the bottom when melted. When water bubbles release from the butter (2-3 minutes) and begin to pop, add eggs. When whites cook to desired firmness, flip eggs and cook on other side to desired firmness. Optional, cover with 8-inch cover and cook to desired firmness.

French Scrambled Eggs

Prepare eggs to scramble by placing 2 eggs in bowl. Add 1 tablespoon of water and whip thoroughly with a whisk or fork.

Preheat 8-inch gourmet Chef Pan over medium heat. Place a small amount of unsalted butter in the pan, enough to cover the bottom when melted. When water bubbles release from butter (2-3 minutes) and begin to pop, add eggs. As eggs begin to cook, draw cooked part from the edge of the pan toward the center with a fork allowing uncooked egg batter to move to hot surface of pan. Repeat process until eggs are scrambled to desired firmness.

Ham & Cheese Omelet

Prepare eggs for omelet by placing 2 eggs in bowl. Add 1 tablespoon of water and whip thoroughly with a whisk or fork.

Preheat 10-inch gourmet Chef Pan over medium heat. Place a small amount of unsalted butter in pan, enough to cover the bottom when melted. When water bubbles release from butter (2-3 minutes) and begin to pop, add the ham, sauté for about 3 minutes. Spread ham evenly.

Add eggs and begin to cook, draw cooked part toward center with a fork allowing uncooked egg batter to move to hot surface of pan. Repeat process until eggs form a disc. Add grated cheese, or other desired ingredients and cook to desired firmness. When done, loosen omelet and fold onto serving plate.

Soft Cooked Eggs

In a cool 1-quart saucepan (1.5 L utensil) place eggs and 2 tablespoons water for one egg, adding 1 tablespoon for each additional egg, up to six. (Use ½ cup (120 ml) water for more than 6 eggs.) Cover pan and open vent. Cook on medium heat until steam appears, about 2 minutes.

For electric range, turn off heat. For gas range, turn flame as low as possible. Time the eggs from the instant steam appears through Vapor Vent. Close vent and continue cooking 3-4 minutes for soft cooked, 5 minutes for very firm white and medium soft yolk.

Hard Cooked Eggs

Use the same method as above, adding additional water for additional eggs. Cover and close the vent. Cook over medium heat for 5 minutes. Turn burner off and leave covered 10 minutes. Cool in cold water, then peel.

Poached Eggs

Pour 1 cup (240 ml) hot water into 1¼-quart Saucepan/Small Skillet with egg poaching rack. Break eggs into lightly buttered egg cups. Place on egg poaching rack. Cover and close the vent. Cook over medium heat until steam appears. Reduce to low. Continue cooking 3-4 minutes for soft cooked eggs, or longer to desired firmness.

Pancakes & Crepes

Prepare pancake batter according to package directions. Preheat 13-inch (33 cm) Chef Pan over medium heat. Place a small amount of unsalted butter in the pan, enough to cover the bottom when melted. When water bubbles release from butter (2-3 minutes) and begin to pop, add pancake batter to pan.

Cook until bubbles appear on top of cake and burst (about 3-5 minutes). Flip pancake and cook the other side until done (about 2-3 minutes). When done, serve with butter and maple syrup.

Crepes can be cooked the same way, only with a much thinner batter.

See videos on How to Cook Perfect Eggs, Omelets and Crepes at www.healthcraft1.com

NUTRITION BASICS

There is increasing evidence that certain foods may help prevent or hinder some types of cancer. While the evidence continues to accumulate, adding these foods to your diet certainly cannot hurt and likely will help.

It is a particularly smart diet strategy. Eating many kinds of fruits and vegetables is sound advice from the American Cancer Society on cancer-proofing your diet. Most experts also recommend cutting down on fats and eating healthy amounts of fiber-the same prescription that experts say reduces heart attack risks. Maintaining your foods' natural goodness by cooking the waterless, greaseless way only makes good sense.

As human beings there are four major factors that influence our health: heredity, the environment, **nutrition**, and the amount and type of **exercise** we get.

We have the most control over our nutrition and the amount of exercise. This section has been designed as a primer on nutrition, to help you find a more healthful way to eat. By understanding where we currently are on the road to better health, we will all live longer more healthful lives.

A quote from the Surgeon General's report on Nutrition and Health focuses on the cultural and social pleasures of our heritage.

Today, 12.5 million children are overweight in the United States—more than 17 percent. Overweight children are at greater risk for many serious health problems. This initiative promotes the importance of healthy eating and physical activity at a young age to help prevent overweight and obesity in this country.

Estimated Total Deaths & Percent of Total Deaths for the 10 Leading Causes of Death in the USA

Rank	Cause of Death	Number	Percent
I	Heart Disease*	652,486	27.7
2	Cancer*	553,888	23.1
3	Strokes*	150,074	6.3
4	Lung Disease	121,987	5.1
5	Unintentional Injuries	112,012	4.7

6	Diabetes mellitus*	73,138	3.1
7	Alzheimer's Disease	65,965	2.8
8	Pneumonia & Influenza	59.664	2.5
9	Kidney Disease*	42,480	1.8
10	Blood Disease Septicemia	33,373	1.4
	All other causes	532,548	22.2
	Total	**2,338,011**	

Source: National Center for Health Statistics, Reports Vol. 56, No. 5 2007
* Causes of death in which diet plays a part.

Food Guide Pyramid

In 1992 the Food and Drug Administration revised the four basic food groups we grew up with expanding it to include nutritional ingredients they believed to be required in our daily diets. Today, with more than 65% of Americans overweight or obese they realize it no longer works and they're making an effort to revise it.

Recent independent and university research on the glycemic index and type-2 diabetes confirms that a diet high in healthy vegetables, lean meat, and low in processed, high-glycemic carbohydrates, has proven to be a more accurate alternative for weight management and better health. The food guide below provides examples to help you in making better choices, and with a nutritional breakdown of every recipe, per serving, it will allow you to prepare healthier meals.

Foods to Focus on...

Healthy Vegetables 4 to 9 servings per day, like; carrots, green beans, broccoli, spinach, asparagus, and other green vegetables, ½ cup cooked or 1 cup raw = 1 serving.

Healthy Proteins 2 to 4 servings per day, like; low-fat cottage cheese, seafood, lean meats and skinless poultry, 3 to 4 ounces or ½ cup = 1 serving. 2 whole eggs or 3 to 4 egg whites.

Healthy Fats 2 to 6 serving per day, like; 1 teaspoon olive oil or sesame seed oil, 2 - 3 tablespoons nuts and seeds, or ¼ avocado.

Healthy Carbohydrates 1 to 4 servings per day, like; pears, apples, dates, oranges, and cherries, milk, plain yogurt, legumes, whole-wheat grain, rice bran, yams, sweet potatoes, and pasta cooked al dente (firm to the bite), ½ cup = 1 serving.

Foods with Some Nutritional Value...

Moderate Carbohydrate Foods 2 to 4 servings per day, like; apricots, papayas, fresh pineapple and raisins, ½ cup = 1 serving.

High Carbohydrate Foods should be limited to 1serving per day like; white rice and breakfast cereals, ½ cup = 1 serving. Choose long grain or brown rice, and whole breakfast cereals.

Foods to Consume Sparingly...

Sugar and sugar based foods, sugar candy, sweets, processed flour baked goods.

Source: Glycemic Index Weight Loss; Lucy Beale and Joan Clark, R.D., C.D.E. pages 68, 69, 70

Thanks to advances in medical research we know about complex carbohydrates, and the difference between processed and unprocessed grains, types of proteins and fats, and how eating too many servings of high-glycemic carbohydrate foods will add our waistlines and decrease our chances for longevity.

This chart replaces the Old Food Guide Pyramid in earlier editions of our cookbook and takes the original food groups and expands them into the recommended categories based on research on the Glycemic Index and what many health-practitioners recommend for a healthy diet.

As always, before beginning any diet, health or weight management program, we suggest you consult with your family doctor.

How many servings do you need?

	Sedentary Women & Older Adults	Children, Teenage Girls, Active Women, Sedentary Men	Teenage Boys, Active Men, Very Active Women
Healthy Vegetables	4	6 to 7	9
Healthy Proteins	2	3	4
Healthy Carbohydrates	1 to 2	3	4
Healthy Fats (tablespoon)	1	2	3
Moderate Carbohydrates	2	3	4
High Carbohydrates	0 to 1	1	1 to 2

What Counts as a Serving?

Breads, Cereal, Rice, Pasta

1 slice bread (1 oz), ½ English muffin, regular bagel or soft pretzel, ½ bun or pita (1 oz), ½ slice firm hearth loaf, ½ oz crackers, cookies or pretzels, ½ medium muffin, 1 small waffle 3 ½" (9 cm) square, 1 pancake 4" (10 cm), ½ cup cooked rice, bulgur, barley, or other whole grain, ½ cup cooked pasta or couscous, 1 oz cold cereal (amount varies, read labels), ½ cup cooked cereal (⅓ uncooked), 2 cups plain popcorn, 1 slice pizza (⅛ of 10" pizza), ½ of 1 flour or corn tortilla (1 oz)

Vegetables

1 cup raw vegetables, carrots, green beans, broccoli, spinach, asparagus, yams, sweet potatoes, and green leafy vegetables; if chopped or cooked ½ cup; ¾ cup vegetable juice, equals 1 serving.

Fruit

1 medium pear, apple, orange or ½ cup if chopped, cooked or canned; ¾ cup fruit juice, equals 1 serving.

Milk, Yogurt, Cheese

½ cup milk, plain yogurt or cottage cheese; 1-2 ounces natural cheese, equals 1 serving.

Meat, Poultry, Fish, Dry Beans, Eggs

3-4 ounces meat, poultry or fish or ½ cup; ½ cup cooked dry beans; 2 whole eggs or 3-4 egg whites; equals 1 serving. 2 tablespoons peanut butter count as 1 oz of meat.

Healthy Fats

1 teaspoon seed oils like olive oil, sesame oil, safflower, sunflower; fish oils; 2-3 tablespoons nuts and seeds, ¼ avocados; equals 1 serving.

Take Control

How do you make a change in your eating habits and take control of your own health? *The American Cancer Society* recommends the following:

Protective Factors

GREEN VEGETABLES, eat more of the crucifers: Brussels-sprouts, broccoli, cauliflower, all cabbages, and kale.

HIGH FIBER FOODS, eat more whole grains, fruits and vegetables, wheat and bran cereals, rice, popcorn, and whole-wheat breads.

VITAMIN A, eat foods with beta-carotene: carrots, peaches, apricots, squash and broccoli.

VITAMIN C, eat fresh fruits and vegetables like grapefruit, cantaloupe, oranges, strawberries, red and green peppers, broccoli and tomatoes.

WEIGHT CONTROL, Control your Weight through regular exercise and sensible eating.

Risk Factors

HIGH-FAT DIET cut fat intake. Eat lean meats, fish, skinned poultry, and reduced fat dairy products. Avoid pastries and candies.

SODIUM AND FOOD PRESERVATIVES, choose these foods only on occasions; bacon, ham, hotdogs, and salt cured-meats and fish.

TOBACO, smoking is the biggest cancer risk of all. Pick a day to quit now.

ALCOHOL is linked to kidney and liver disease. If you drink, do so in moderation.

EXCESSIVE SUN exposure can cause skin cancer and other damage. Protect yourself.

Reduce Your Risk of Cancer

Make a commitment to yourself today to make healthy food choices. Choose foods high in vitamin A, vitamin C, and fiber and consume more cruciferous vegetables; broccoli, cauliflower, brussel sprouts, cabbage.

Foods high in vitamin A may help protect against cancers of the esophagus, larynx, and lung. Choose squash, apricot, and spinach. Fresh foods are the best source of beta-carotene, not vitamin pills. Likewise, vitamin C may help protect against cancers of the esophagus and stomach and is found naturally in many fresh foods and vegetables. Adding high fiber may protect you against colon cancer and cruciferous (the cabbage family type) appear to protect against colon, stomach, and respiratory cancers.

Why We Cook

> To make food more palatable and appetizing
> To kill harmful bacteria on food
> To make food more digestible
> To entertain, be creative, and have fun

Keep in mind, however, a wide selection of foods are available in our modern day world, what we do with them prior to consumption either adds or subtracts from their nutritional value and to our health.

Dietary Intake

The following shows the current percentages of average dietary intake in the United States. As you can see, in this country complex carbohydrate consumption is a mere 58% of what it should be. The same is true for sugar consumption only reversed. We eat more, not less, sugar than we should and out fat intake skyrockets.

Current Levels

> Complex Carbohydrates 28%
> Unsaturated Fat 19%
> Refined Sugars 18%
> Saturated Fat 16%
> Protein 12%
> Polyunsaturated Fat 7%

Recommended Levels

> Complex Carbohydrates 54%
> Protein 16%
> Unsaturated Fat 5%
> Refined Sugars 5%
> Saturated Fat 5%
> Polyunsaturated Fat 5%

Suggestions:
>Eat a variety of foods
>Maintain desirable weight
>Avoid too much fat, saturated fat, and cholesterol
>Eat foods with adequate starch and fiber
>Avoid too much sugar
>Avoid too much sodium
>If you drink alcoholic beverages, do so in moderation

Carbohydrates provide 4 calories per gram
Proteins provide 4 calories per gram
Fat provides over twice as many, 9 to 11 calories per gram

Basics on Metabolism

Metabolism is the process by which food is converted into useful energy. This begins with a chemical processes in gastrointestinal tract changing plant an animal food into less complex components so they can be absorbed to fulfill their various functions in the body; growth, repair and fuel. The body gets its energy in the form of carbohydrates, protein and fats. We measure the energy available in foods, and the energy needed for metabolism, physical activity and digestion, as calories.

Carbohydrates provide 4 calories per gram, Proteins provide 4 calories per gram, and Fats provide 9 to 11 calories per gram. The daily caloric need varies widely and is dependent upon height, weight, age, level of activity, state of health, and heredity as well. It is generally accepted that the "typical" adult woman needs 1,500 – 1,800 calories per day, and the "typical" adult man needs 2,000 - 3,000 calories per day.

Each pound of human body fat has about 3,500 calories of energy. Body fat is converted into energy when the calorie intake in food is inadequate. Likewise, calories eaten in excess of need are stored as body fat. A pound of body fat can be lost in one week by reducing energy intake by 500 calories per day, or by increasing physical activity by 500 calories per day. A combination of decreased intake and increased output will lead to a recommended slow healthy weight loss of 2 pounds per week, allowing the body's metabolism and past eating habits to change gradually towards permanent weight loss.

Fats are stored in the body and used as a later energy source. The body's metabolism is a very complex process, and some fat must be included in our diet for important body functions including; insulation, transportation of fat soluble vitamins, i.e.

Vitamin A is essential for vision, cell growth and development, reproduction, a strong immune system, healthy hair, skin and mucous membranes.

Vitamin D is essential for proper metabolism of calcium for strong bones.

Vitamin E is essential for healthy nerve function and reproduction.

Vitamin K is essential for clotting of blood.

Metabolic Facts

Fat calories are deposited as body fat, whereas carbohydrates are more likely to be burned as body heat, for example: eating 100 calories of pretzels (carbohydrates) result in 25 calories being used for digestion and processing and 75 calories left to be stored; eating 100 calories of salad dressing (fat) results in 3 to 5 calories used for digestion with 95 to 97 calories being stored.

Fatty acids in the small intestine are passively absorbed, using no calories; carbohydrates and proteins both require calories in their digestive process.

Eating fats with sugar may create increased obesity because sugar simulates the release of insulin which encourages excessive fat storage.

Extremely low-fat diets (less than 20 percent of total calories in fat) will not necessarily cause weight loss because the individual may eat excessive calories from other sources.
We need to aim towards a healthy ratio of body fat and lean muscle mass which is 15 to 20 percent body fat for men and 19 to 24 percent for women.

In the muscle, fat is only burned for fuel in the presence of oxygen and carbohydrates. Include a regular moderate level aerobic exercise to increase oxidation of stored body fat.

To have adequate nutritional intake and lower fat — have at least five servings of vegetables a day and exercise 30 minutes five times per week.

Lower Fat Calorie Intake. Reaching and maintaining a healthier weight is important for your overall health and well being. If you are significantly overweight, you have a greater risk of developing many diseases including high blood pressure, Type 2 diabetes, stroke, and some forms of cancer. For obese adults, even losing a few pounds or preventing further weight gain has health benefits.

Reaching a healthier weight is a balancing act. The secret is learning how to balance your "energy in" and "energy out" over the long run.

"Energy in" is the calories from the foods and beverages you have each day. "Energy out" is the calories you burn for basic body functions and physical activity.

Maintaining Weight, Your weight will stay the same when the calories you eat and drink equal the calories you burn.

Losing Weight, You will lose weight when the calories you eat and drink are less than the calories you burn.

Gaining Weight, You will gain weight when the calories you eat and drink are greater than the calories you burn.

Understand & Use Food Labels

The new Food Label format should make food shopping much easier for everyone. It will be especially helpful for those who need to limit certain nutrients due to illness, disease prevention and for healthy weight loss. To follow along, take a packaged or box food out of your pantry.

The food label also carries an up-to-date easier-to-use nutritional guide, and is required on most all packaged foods. It serves as a key to help in planning a healthy diet.

1. The title, **Nutrition Facts,** signals that the label contains the required information.

2. **Serving Size** is now consistent across all food product lines, stating both the Serving Size in metric measurement and the amount of **Servings per Container.**

3. **Amount per Serving** indicates the total Calories per serving. Calories from Fat per serving are also listed. For a healthy diet it is recommended that you consume no more than 30% calories from fat on a daily basis.

4. **% Daily Values** indicates how a food fits into the recommended daily diet for 2,000 calories.

5. The **List of Nutrients** covers those most important to the health of today's consumer. The food's producer may also include information about Vitamins and Minerals. Foods that contain a minimal amount of nutrients, required on the standard label, can use a short label format and not include this information. This may also be the case with food products in very small packages and cans.

6. **Percent Daily Values**, in the small print at the bottom of the label, are maximums, as with fat (less than 65g); others are minimums, as with Total de Carbohydrates (300 grams or more). The daily values on the label are based on a daily diet of 2,000 and 2,500 calories. Individuals should adjust the values to fit their desired calorie intake.

7. The label also indicates the number of **calories per gram of Fat, Carbohydrate, and Protein.** The numbers are rounded off.

Of the six items shown in bold print on the label, four – namely Calories, Total Fat, Cholesterol, and Sodium, will alert consumers to the items they should consumer in moderation. Saturated Fat values are also provided.

More on Food Labels

Another advantage of understanding and using Food Labels is the requirement of standardized portions per servings. In the past, food manufacturers could alter the content of their products by juggling the Serving Size. For example, in order to make potato chips appear to be low calorie, low fat, and low sodium, the serving size was two chips, and the amounts were usually given in ounces or other weights not commonly understood by the public. The new regulations now mandate portion sizes that are more typical of the amounts people actually consume, and are now listed in common measurements.

Daily Values (DV) and Percent of Daily Values also provide another nutritional content indicator. The Daily Values are the reference numbers set by the government and are based on current nutritional recommendations, and correlated with healthy diets of 2,000 or 2,500 calories, referenced on the bottom of the label.

Food Component DV for all Calorie Levels

Cholesterol	300 mg
Sodium	2,400 mg
Potassium*	3,500 mg
*Optional on Nutrition label	

The Percent of Daily Values (%DV) gives a general idea as to the food's nutrient contributions to the 2,000 calorie reference diet. In all cases you must remember that you may need more than 2,000 calories per day.

Guidelines for Percentages of Daily Values

Food Component	Calculated as*
Total fat	30% of total calories
Saturated fat	10% of total calories
Total Carbohydrate	60% of total calories
Dietary Fiber	11.5 gm/1000 calories
Protein**	10% of total calories

*Numbers may be rounded for labeling

**% Daily Values for protein is optional

In order to build a healthful diet using these concepts and different calorie levels, use the Daily Nutrient Chart below to find the nutrient amounts and total Percentage Daily Value indicated for your calorie choice level. This will help you to compare foods and make informed, healthier choices.

Daily Nutrient Needs for Different Calorie Levels*

Food Component	1,600	2,000**	2,200	2,500	2,800	3,200
Total Fat (g)	53	65	73	80	93	107
Saturated Fat (g)	18	20	24	25	31	36
Total Carbohy-drate	240	300	330	375	420	480
Dietary Fiber (g)	20***	25	25	30	32	37
Protein	46****	50	55	64	70	80

Your total **% Daily Value** for each of these nutrients in all the foods you eat in one day can add up to:

80%	100%	110%	125%	140%	160%

- **Numbers*** may be rounded
- **% Daily Value**** on the label for total fat, saturated fat, carbohydrate, dietary fiber, and protein (if listed is based on a 2,000 calorie reference diet.)
- **20 g**** is the minimum amount of fiber recommended for all calorie levels below 1,800. Source: National Cancer Institute.
- **46 g****** is the minimum amount of protein recommended for all calorie levels below 1,800. Source: Recommended Dietary Allowances 1989.

NOTE: These calorie levels may not apply to children and adolescents who have varying caloric requirements. For specific advice concerning calorie levels, please consult a registered dietitian, qualified health professional, or pediatrician.

Food Label Legislation

Another positive aspect of food labeling legislation is it eliminated nutrient content claims that were not valid. The label format mandates criteria for definition of food claims such as Fat Free, High Fiber, Low Calorie, etc.

Label Claim	Definitions
Calorie free	less than 5 calories
Low calorie	40 calories of less
Light or Lite	one-third fewer calories of 50% less fat
Fat free	less than ½ gram fat
Low fat	3 grams or less, fat
Cholesterol free	less than 2 mg cholesterol and 2 gm or less saturated fat
Low cholesterol	20 mg or less cholesterol and 2 mg or less saturated fat
Sodium free	less than 5 mg sodium
Very low sodium	35 mg or less
Low sodium	140 mg or less
High fiber	5 grams or more

It's anticipated that new definition will be developed by food manufacturers identifying other nutrients needing clarification.

An area of considerable controversy has developed regarding the use of health claims on food packaging. A health claim is defined as a label statement describing the relationship between a nutrient and disease or health-related condition. The food must meet specific nutrient levels if it is to be allowed to make a health claim. Currently, seven types of health claims are allowed.

Nutrient-Disease Relationship
- Diet high in calcium reduces the risk of osteoporosis
- Diet high in fiber-containing grains, fruits, and vegetables reduces the risk of cancer.
- Diet high in fruits or vegetables is high dietary fiber or vitamin A or C reduces risks of cancer.

- Diet high in fiber from fruits, vegetables, and grain products reduces the risk of heart disease.
- Diet low in fat reduces risks of cancer.
- Diet low in saturated fat and cholesterol reduces risk of heart disease.
- Diet low in sodium reduces risk of high blood pressure.

Food labels are required on all canned and packaged foods except:

- Foods produced by companies with food sales of less than $50,000 per year.
- Restaurant food
- Food prepared for immediate consumption, such as airplane meals
- Food sold by food service vendors
- Food sold in bulk bins
- Plain coffee, tea, spices, and other foods without significant amounts of nutrients

There is a great deal of excellent label information available to the general public through organizations such as the National Food Processors Association, The American Diabetics Association and the manufacturers of the individual products. As with most things in our lives the more you know about food labels the more freedom you will have in developing healthful meals. Never-the-less, your best prospect for living a healthy life style is to choose fresh foods.

The Point System

Calorie Points are a simplified way of counting calories. This is the best system for people who want to lose, maintain or gain weight. Many diabetics use the Point System to assist in managing their disease.

Calorie Points may be used to count several nutrients in addition to calories. The nutrients include, but are not limited to sodium, carbohydrate, fiber, protein, and potassium. Using the points makes it easy to manage a healthy diet.

The more traditional method of counting calories is time consuming, and not as accurate as most people believe. Calorie values published in different books vary as does the calorie content of the foods. For example; there may be many calorie differences in the same size apples growing on opposite sides of the same tree. Although counting calories is not an exact science, the lists of nutrients are the best tool available.

Definitions of Points
The nutrients considered have assigned point values as follows:

> A Calorie Point is 75 calories abbreviated as (CAL)
> A Carbohydrate Point is 15 grams of Carbohydrate abbreviated as (CHO)
> A Fiber Point is 2 grams of Dietary Fiber abbreviated as (FIB)
> A Sodium Point is 23 milligrams of Sodium abbreviated as (NA)
> A Cholesterol Point is 10 milligrams of Cholesterol abbreviated as (CHOL)
> A Protein Point is 8 grams of Protein abbreviated as (PRO)

The recipes listed and analyzed in this cookbook for Health Craft by Dr. Ann Hunter provide nutrient values and points for the six selected nutrients.

Counting 20 calorie points instead of 1,500 calories is one example of the simplicity of the calorie point system.

Calorie/Carbohydrate Point Conversions
The first two columns of the chart below list calories and the conversion values in points. Remember, a Calorie Point is equal to about 75 calories. The third column is the grams of carbohydrate suggested for each calorie level and its conversion to carbohydrate points shown in the fourth column. The final columns represent fat calories and fat grams. It is now easier to count fat as grams because that value is found on all food labels. Example; For a 1,500 calorie plan you would want to consume 20 calorie points, 11 carbohydrate points, and 42 grams of fat.

Calories	Points	Grams of Carbohydrates 55% of Total Calories	Carbohydrate Points	Fat 25% of Total Calories	Fat Grams
1,200	16	660	9	300	33
1,300	17 ½	715	9 ½	325	36
1,400	18 ½	770	10	350	39
1,500	20	825	11	375	42
1,600	21 ½	880	12	400	44
1,700	22 ½	935	12 ½	425	47
1,800	24	990	13	450	50
1,900	25 ½	1,045	14	475	53
2,000	26 ½	1,100	14 ½	500	56
2,100	28	1,155	15	525	58
2,200	29 ½	1,210	16	550	61
2,300	31	1,265	17	575	64
2,400	32	1,320	17 ½	600	67
2,500	33 ½	1,375	18	625	69
2,600	35	1,430	19	650	72
2,700	36	1,485	20	675	75
2,800	37 ½	1,540	20 ½	700	78
2,900	38 ½	1,595	21	725	81
3,000	40	1,650	22	750	83
4,000	53	2,200	29	1,000	111
5,000	67	2,75	36 ½	1,250	139

Fiber Points

Because of the health benefits of including dietary fiber in your diet, we suggest that you count dietary fiber points as well. Ten (10) fiber points per day are recommended for the first two-week period. Fifteen (15) fiber points per day are recommended for the second two weeks. Increase the maximum to 20-25 fiber points per day, as tolerated.

The Issue of Control

A truly successful eating plan is one that is safe, healthy, and allows you to eat the foods you enjoy. To succeed, you must stay on the new plan until you have modified your harmful behaviors and gained control over your eating habits. The plan is a success when you reach your goal and maintain that new weight. It is best to think of this activity as learning to eat properly rather than being on a diet.

Nine Points to Assist in Control

1. Do not adopt a plan so low in calories that you can't get the needed nutrients and your body slows down leading to decreased calorie burn. A rule of thumb is at least 1,200 calories for females and 1,500 for males.

    A dietitian or your family doctor can compute the calorie level that will allow you to lose weight safely. (Factors such as repeated dieting may result in reduced metabolic rate requiring fewer calories than indicated on the following chart.)

Find your weight range and activity level. Multiply your actual weight by the calories per pound shown under your activity level.

Weight If Overweight	Sedentary Activity	Light to Moderate Activity	Very Active
up to 200 lbs	12	13	15
201 to 250	10	11	12 to 13
251 to 300	9	10	11
300 lbs and over	8	9	10
If normal weight	12	14	16 to 18

SEDENTARY ACTIVITY – Most of the day is spent in activities such as TV, reading, handwork, etc.

LIGHT TO MODERATE ACTIVITY – Most of the day is spent in activities such as walking, housework, golf, etc.

VERY ACTIVE – Most of the day is spent in activities such as walking briskly, yard work, scrubbing floors, dancing, etc., or a regular exercise program is scheduled.

2. Eat at least three to five smaller meals a day and a snack if desired. These must be within the allowed calories and fat grams. This plan keeps you from getting too hungry and, therefore, out of control.

3. Do not weigh yourself more than once a week. Remember that a 1-2 pound weight loss per week or 4-10 pounds per month will be the most healthful and permanent loss.

4. Take the time to identify current bad habits and create ways to overcome them.

5. Write down the foods eaten and point values for the nutrients you are counting. Writing the items down is the only way to keep track of intake for the first few months.

6. Exercise daily to improve your calorie burn, muscle tone, body configuration, raise your metabolic rate, improve your mental attitude, and relieve stress.

7. Don't let a binge become an excuse to quit. Start on the eating plan again.

8. Special occasions and foods can be worked into your eating plan.

9. It is essential that you have a well balanced, adequate nutrient intake. Refer to information on the Food Guide Pyramid page. For your basic nutritional needs.

Calorie, Carbohydrate & Sodium Conversion Chart

The following charts are provided to help you determine points from label information.

Calorie Conversion Chart		Carbohydrate Conversion Chart	
Calorie Content On Label	Calorie Point	Carbohydrate Content On Label	Carbohydrate Points
19-56	½	4-11	½
57-94	1	12-19	1
95-131	1 ½	20-26	1 ½
132-169	2	27-34	2
170-206	2 ½	35-41	2 ½
207-244	3	42-49	3
245-281	3 ½	50-56	3 ½
282-319	4	57-64	4
320-356	4 ½	65-71	4 ½
357-394	5	72-79	5
395-431	5 ½	80-86	5 ½
432-469	6	87-94	6
470-506	6 ½	95-101	6 ½

507-544	7	102-109	7
545-581	7 ½	110-116	7 ½
582-619	8	117-124	8
620-656	8 ½	125-131	8 ½
657-694	9	132-139	9
695-731	9 ½	140-146	9 ½
732-769	10	147-154	10
770-806	10 ½		
807-844	11		

Sodium Conversion Chart

Sodium Content On Label	Sodium Points
13-33	1
34-56	2
57-79	3
80-102	4
103-125	5
126-148	6
149-171	7
172-194	8
195-217	9
218-240	10
333-355	15
448-480	20
563-595	25
678-710	30

Sample Menu for 1500 Calories

A sample menu has been included to help give you ideas for planning. The example includes a cookie to show you that all "fun" do not become things of the past. People with more strict needs would have to modify this sample.

		20 Calorie Points	11 Carbs Points	10-20 Fiber Points	42 Fat Grams
Breakfast					
Cornflakes	1 cup	1.5	1.5	1.5	0
Banana	½	1	1	1	0
Whole wheat toast	1 slice	1	1	1	1
Margarine	1 teaspoon	.5	0	0	0
Milk, ½% fat	1 ½ cups	1.5	1.5	0	0
Lunch					
Whole wheat bread	2 slices	2	2	2	2.5
Turkey	2 ounces	1	0	0	7.5
Cheese	¾ ounce	1	0	0	1
Salad dressing	½ tablespoon	.5	0	0	1
Carrot sticks	6 to 8	0	0	.5	0
Oatmeal chocolate Chip cookie	1	1	.5	1	2.5
Snack					
Whole wheat crackers	2	1	1	1	0
Peanut butter	1 tablespoon	1.5	.5	.5	2.5
Dinner					
Lean roast beef	2 ounces	2	0	0	10
Baked potato	1	2	2	2	0
Margarine	2 teaspoons	1	0	0	10
Green beans	½ cup	0	0	1	0
Spinach salad	½ cup	0	0	2.5	0
Dressing	1 tablespoon	1	0	0	0
Strawberries	¼ cup	.5	.5	1	0
		20	**11.5**	**15**	**41**

Appetizers, Soups & Salads...

Chickpea Soup with Cumin and Cilantro

Sopa de Garbanzos
Serves 6
Preparation Time: 40 minutes
Equipment: French chef knife, Kitchen Machine food cutter, 3-quart saucepan, blender

1½	cups cooked chickpeas
1	onion, coarsely chopped, #3 French fry blade
1½	teaspoons cumin seeds, ground fine
4	cups (1 L) low sodium or homemade beef or chicken stock
1	tablespoon flour
3	tablespoons unsalted butter
½	cup (120 ml) light cream,* or half and half
	Sea salt or kosher salt & pepper to taste (optional)
2	tablespoons cilantro, chopped

In the 3-quart (3 L) saucepan combine chickpeas, onion, cumin, and chicken stock. Bring to a slow boil. Reduce heat and simmer for 20 minutes. Puree the mixture in a blender on low speed and return to the pan.

In a mixing bowl, make a paste by mixing flour and 2 tablespoons softened butter and add to the soup mix in small amounts at a time. After each addition, whisk until smooth. Simmer over low heat for 10 minutes.

Add the remaining 1 tablespoon of butter (optional) and whisk to combine. Add salt (optional) and pepper to taste.

To serve, ladle into individual soup bowls and top with cilantro.

> NOTE: To reduce fat, omit cream and 1 tablespoon butter (butter and cream are included in nutritional breakdown).

NUTRITIONAL BREAKDOWN PER SERVING: Calories 220; Fat Grams 14; Carbohydrate grams 17; Cholesterol mg 25; Sodium mg 266.

THE POINT SYSTEM: Calorie Points 3; Protein Points 1; Fat Grams 14; Sodium Points 12; Fiber Points 2; Carbohydrate Points 1; Cholesterol Points 3.

Poppy Seed Fruit Salad

Serves 5
Preparation Time: 15 minutes
Equipment: French chef knife, 2-quart stainless mixing bowl, 1-quart stainless mixing bowl

1	10½ ounce (300 g) can mandarin orange
1	8 ounce (230 g) can pineapple tidbits, or
½	fresh pineapple, cubed
1½	cup small strawberries or seedless fresh grapes
1	medium apple, cored and cubed
½	cup pineapple yogurt
½	teaspoon poppy seeds
	Lettuce leaves

Drain mandarin oranges; drain pineapple, reserving 1 tablespoon juice. If using strawberries, cut in half. Mix all fruit in a 2-quart mixing bowl. Toss lightly to mix.

For dressing, in the 1-quart mixing bowl stir together yogurt, poppy seeds and reserved pineapple juice.

To serve, line salad plates with lettuce leaves. Arrange fruit mixture on lettuce. Drizzle with dressing over fruit.

NUTRITIONAL BREAKDOWN PER SERVING: Calories 101; Fat Grams 1; Carbohydrate Grams 23; Protein Grams 2; Cholesterol mg 1; Sodium mg 16.

THE POINT SYSTEM: Calorie Points 1½; Protein Points 0; Fat Grams 1; Sodium Points ½; Fiber Points 1; Carbohydrate Points 1½; Cholesterol Points 0.

Thai Grilled Sirloin Salad

Serves 8
Preparation Time: 45 minutes
Equipment: French chef knife, Kitchen Machine food cutter, large skillet,
3-quart stainless mixing bowl

1	teaspoon pepper, freshly ground
1	pound (460 g) beef sirloin, trimmed
1	small head red cabbage, shredded blade #5
1	head romaine lettuce cut in 1 inch (2.5 cm) strips
½	cup mint leaves
2	shallots, peeled and thinly sliced into rings
8	green onions, chopped
2	hot peppers, seeded and diced
1	cup chicken broth or stock
1	teaspoon fresh lime juice
2	tablespoons fish sauce
1	teaspoon sugar
1	teaspoon roasted rice powder (See page 205)

Preheat skillet over medium-high heat. While the pan is heating, rub black pepper into beef sirloin. Place sirloin in skillet, when it loosens from the pan (about 4-5 minutes), turn and sear about 3 minutes on other side (beef should be rare). Remove sirloin to platter, and place in freezer 30-45 minutes. Note: slightly freezing will make sirloin easier to slice thinly. Drain excess fat from skillet and place on the side, do not clean.

While beef is cooling, in the mixing bowl combine cabbage, romaine lettuce, mint, shallots, green onions and hot peppers.

Slice sirloin thin across the grain. Reheat skillet over medium-high heat. When the skillet begins to sizzle deglaze with chicken stock. Add lime juice, fish sauce, sugar and rice powder, stir and bring to a simmer. Add sliced sirloin and remove skillet from heat. Let cool for 3-5 minutes and pour over prepared salad and toss well. Serve with soy sauce if desired.

NUTRIONAL BREAKDOWN PER SERVING: Calories 113; Fat Grams 3; Carbohydrate Grams 8; Protein Grams 13; Cholesterol mg 44; Sodium mg 469 (230 if homemade chicken stock).

THE POINT SYSTEM: Calorie Points 1 ½; Protein Points 2; Fat Grams 3; Sodium Points 20 (10 if homemade chicken stock); Fiber Points 1; Carbohydrate Points ½; Cholesterol Points 4.

German Potato Salad

Serves: 6-8
Yields 4 cups
Preparation Time: 30 minutes
Equipment: French chef knife, cutting board, Kitchen Machine
food cutter, large skillet, slotted spoon.

2	strips bacon, sliced or Canadian bacon
5	potatoes, waffle cut blade #5
1	onion, chopped blade #3
¼	cup (60 ml) vinegar (white distilled or apple cider vinegar)
2	tablespoons raw sugar (optional, 1 tablespoon sugar)

In the skillet, cook bacon over medium heat until slightly crisp. Remove from pan with a slotted spoon and set aside.

Add potatoes and onions to skillet, cover, close the vent and reduce heat to medium-low and sauté about 10 minutes. With a flexible spatula, turn potatoes, cover, and continue cooking, about 5-7 minutes.

Combine vinegar and sugar; add mixture to pan along with crumbled bacon.

Serve as a side dish with Baby Back Ribs page 101.

NUTRITIONAL BREAKDOWN PER SERVING: Calories 168; Fat Grams 2; Carbohydrate Grams 34; Protein Grams 4; Cholesterol mg 3; Sodium mg 71.

THE POINT SYSTEM: Calorie Points 2; Protein Points 0; Fat Points 2; Sodium Points 3; Fiber Points 1; Carbohydrate Points 2 ½; Cholesterol Points 0.

Orange Cucumber Salad

Serves: 4
Preparation Time: 10 minutes
Equipment: Kitchen Machine food cutter, French chef knife,
cutting board, 2-quart mixing bowl

1	cucumber, sliced blade #4, or waffle cut blade #5
1	11 ounce (310 g) can mandarin orange sections drained
1	small green pepper, chopped (½ cup)
2	tablespoons parsley, chopped
½	cup plain yogurt
¼	teaspoon ground thyme
	Salad greens

In mixing bowl, combine cucumber, oranges, green pepper, parsley and toss. Combine yogurt and thyme and spoon over salad mixture. Toss lightly, cover, and chill.

Serve with crisp salad greens.

NUTRITIONAL BREAKDOWN PER SERVING: Calories 46; Fat Grams 0; Carbohydrate Grams 9; Protein Grams 3; Cholesterol mg 1; Sodium mg 157.

THE POINT SYSTEM: Calorie Points ½; Protein Points ½; Fat Grams 0; Sodium Points 7; Fiber Points ½; Carbohydrate Points ½; Cholesterol Points 0.

Wedding Soup

Serves: 8
Preparation Time: 40 minutes
Equipment: French chef knife, cutting Board, 2-quart mixing bowl, medium skillet,
4-quart stockpot.

MEATBALLS
½	pound (230 g) extra lean ground beef
1	teaspoon fresh basil, chopped
2	cloves garlic, minced
2	tablespoons tomato paste or ketchup
½	cup Italian bread crumbs
1	egg

SOUP
8	cups chicken broth or homemade chicken stock
3	eggs, beaten
1	cup Pastina (tiny stars) pasta
4	cups whole fresh spinach leaves

In mixing bowl, combine beef, basil, garlic, tomato paste, bread crumbs and egg, mix well and form into (16-20) small meatballs.

Preheat skillet over medium heat and brown meatballs. Remove with a slotted spoon to paper towel to drain.

In 4-quart, add chicken stock and bring to a boil over medium-high heat, then stir in eggs. Add pasta, reduce heat to medium, and simmer until pasta is cooked.

To serve, place 3-4 meatballs in individual soup bowls, add spinach leaves and pour soup mixture into bowl.

NUTRITIONAL BREAKDOWN PER SERVING: Calories 167; Fat Grams 8; Carbohydrate Grams 12; Protein Grams 12; Cholesterol mg 130; Sodium mg 230 (155 with homemade chicken stock).

THE POINT SYSTEM: Calorie Points 2; Protein Points 2; Fat Grams 8; Sodium Points 10 (7 with homemade chicken stock); Fiber Points ½; Carbohydrate Points 1; Cholesterol Points 13.

Chinese Salad

Serves: 10
Preparation Time: 25-30 minutes
Equipment: Kitchen Machine food cutter, French chef knife, cutting board,
10-inch Chef Pan, 1-quart saucepan, large salad serving bowl.

2	tablespoons unsalted butter or low-fat margarine
2	3 ounce (85 g) packages Ramen noodles, crushed
¼	cup sliced almonds
1	tablespoon sesame seeds
¼	cup vinegar (white distilled or apple cider)
½	cup sugar
¼	cup (60 ml) sesame or olive oil
2	tablespoons low sodium soy sauce
1	head Napa cabbage, chopped blade #3
1	bunch green onions, chopped

In 10-inch chef pan melt butter over medium heat. Add Ramen noodles, almonds, and sesame seeds. Brown slowly. Set aside to cool.

In 1-quart saucepan combine vinegar, sugar, oil and soy sauce and bring to a simmer over medium heat. Remove from heat and set aside.

To serve, place chopped cabbage and onion is salad serving bowl. Add cooled Ramen noodle mixture and dressing. Toss and serve.

NUTRIONAL BREAKDOWN PER SERVING: Calories 214; Fat Grams 13; Carbohydrate Grams 23; Protein Grams 5; Cholesterol Grams 13; Sodium Grams 331.

THE POINT SYSTEM: Calorie Points 3; Protein Points 1; Fat Grams 13; Sodium Points 14; Fiber Points 2; Carbohydrate Points 1½; Cholesterol Points 1.

Layer Salad

Serves: 10
Preparation Time: 25-30 minutes
Equipment: French chef knife, cutting board, Kitchen Machine food cutter

1	head lettuce of choice, torn into bite size pieces
8	ounce (230 g) frozen peas, thawed and drained
1	red onion sliced thin, or julienne cut blade #2
3	teaspoons raw sugar (or sugar substitute)
8	ounces (230 g) Swiss cheese, shredded blade #3
½	cup plain nonfat yogurt
½	cup nonfat mayonnaise

In a large glass salad bowl layer prepared ingredients in 3 layers, first layer of lettuce, then one-third portion onions spread evenly, sprinkle 1 teaspoon of sugar over onions, add one-third portion of peas and one-third portion of Swiss cheese. Repeat layer twice more. Combine yogurt and mayonnaise and spread evenly over top.

Salad may be kept in refrigerator for 24 hours before serving.

To serve, toss well to blend ingredients.

NUTRIONAL BREAKDOWN PER SERVING: Calories 126; Fat Grams 6; Carbohydrate Grams 8; Protein Grams 9; Cholesterol Grams 21; Sodium Grams 97.

THE POINT SYSTEM: Calorie Points 1½; Protein Points 1; Fat Grams 6; Sodium Points 4; Fiber Points ½; Carbohydrate Points ½; Cholesterol Points 2.

Chinese Beef-Noodle Soup

Serves: 12

Preparation Time: 2 ½ hours

Equipment: French chef knife, cutting board, Kitchen Machine, 6-quart stockpot, 4-quart stockpot

2 ½	pounds (1.2 kg) beef short ribs, trimmed
7	cups (1.7 kg) water
¼	cup (60 ml) low sodium soy sauce
¼	cup (60 ml) dry sherry
I	tablespoon raw sugar (or sugar substitute)
6	slices fresh ginger, sliced blade #4
8	green onions, chopped
4	cloves garlic, chopped
I	teaspoon aniseed
¼	teaspoon dried hot red pepper flakes
2	turnips, (peeled if waxed) cut into ¼ inch cubes
6	ounces (180 g) egg noodles or rice noodles

In 6-quart stockpot (6 L) combine ribs, water, soy sauce, sherry, and sugar. Bring to boil, skim off froth. Add ginger, half of green onions, garlic, aniseed, and pepper flakes. Reduce heat to low, cover with vent open, and simmer two hours.

Remove from heat. Cool 30 minutes. Remove ribs with slotted spoon. Chop meat, discarding fat and bones. Strain broth through fine sieve into smaller 4-quart stockpot, and add chopped meat. Skim fat or, if time permits, refrigerate and lift fat from surface. Add turnips to broth, simmer covers with vent open 10 minutes, add noodles, and simmer for 7-10 minutes or until done.

To serve, ladle into serving bowl and top with chopped green onions.

NUTRIONAL BREAKDOWN PER SERVING: Calories 234; Fat Grams 6; Carbohydrate Grams 7; Protein Grams 23; Cholesterol Grams 59; Sodium Grams 256.

THE POINT SYSTEM: Calorie Points 3; Protein Points 3; Fat Grams 6; Sodium Points 11; Fiber Points 0; Carbohydrate Points ½; Cholesterol Points 6.

French Onion Soup

Serves: 6

Preparation Time: 1 hour 15 minutes

Equipment: French chef knife, cutting board, 4-quart stockpot

8	onions (Vidalia)
6	cloves garlic, chopped
1	tablespoon unsalted butter or margarine
1	tablespoon oil
6	cups chicken broth or homemade chicken stock
½	cup burgundy wine
6	slices French bread, ¼ inch thick
1	cup Monterey Jack, mozzarella or Swiss cheese

In 4-quart stockpot (4 L), over medium heat, caramelize onion and garlic in butter and oil until translucent and creamy, approximately 30 minutes. Add chicken stock and burgundy wine. Reduce heat and simmer with cover on and vent open 30 minutes.

While soup is simmering, toast French bread in toaster or oven until light brown and dry.

Ladle soup into broil safe bowls. Place one slice of bread on top, cover with mixed cheese, and broil until cheese melts and begins to brown.

NUTRIONAL BREAKDOWN PER SERVING: Calories 337; Fat Grams 15; Carbohydrate Grams 42; Protein Grams 18; Cholesterol Grams 30; Sodium Grams 432 (277 if homemade chicken stock).

THE POINT SYSTEM: Calorie Points 5; Protein Points 2; Fat Grams 15; Sodium Points 19 (11 if homemade chicken stock); Fiber Points 2; Carbohydrate Points 3; Cholesterol Points 3.

Pinto Bean Soup

Serves: 12

Preparation Time: 1 hour 30 minutes

Equipment: Kitchen Machine food cutter, French chef knife, cutting board, 6-quart stockpot

1	pound (460 g) dried pinto beans
3	medium onions, chopped fine blade #2
5	cloves garlic, minced
1	tablespoon olive oil
2	red bell peppers, chopped
1	tablespoon chili powder
2	teaspoons ground cumin
6	cups (1.5 L) water
½	pound (230 g) chorizo (optional)
1	32 ounce (920 g) can tomatoes, chopped, or 2½ lbs fresh plum tomatoes skinned, seeded and chopped
2	cups (489 ml) chicken broth or homemade chicken stock
2	tablespoons tomato paste
2	fresh limes, juice of
½	cup cilantro, chopped

Rinse and pick over beans. Soak overnight in 2 inches (5 cm) water (or rinse beans, cover with water and bring to a boil 2 minutes, remove from heat and let soak 1 hour),

In 6-quart stockpot (6 L) sauté onions and garlic in olive oil until softened, add red peppers, chili powder and cumin.

Drain soaked beans and add to stockpot with 6 cups (1.5 L) water. Cover, open vent, and reduce to low heat 1 hour. If using chorizo, brown and drain on paper towels. Add chorizo, tomatoes, chicken stock and tomato paste to soup, simmer 20-30 minutes or until heated through.

To serve, add 1 teaspoon of lime juice to individual serving bowls, ladle soup into bowls, and top with cilantro.

NUTRIONAL BREAKDOWN PER SERVING: Calories 133; Fat Grams 10; Carbohydrate Grams 20; Protein Grams 12; Cholesterol Grams 5; Sodium Grams 351 (178 if homemade chicken stock and fresh tomatoes).

THE POINT SYSTEM: Calorie Points 2; Protein Points 1½; Fat Grams 10; Sodium Points 15 (9 if homemade stock and fresh tomatoes); Fiber Points 2; Carbohydrate Points 1½; Cholesterol Points ½.

Roasted Red Pepper Salad

Serves: 12
Preparation Time: 1 hour 20 minutes
Equipment: French chef knife, cutting board, large skillet

6	red peppers cut in half cored and seeded
6	tablespoons (90 ml) olive oil
2	tablespoons red wine vinegar
1	clove garlic, chopped
1	green onion, sliced

Flatten red pepper halves with masher or palm of your hand. Preheat skillet over medium-high heat. Brush skin of peppers with olive oil. Place skin side down in hot skillet, occasionally pressing peppers flat with masher or spatula to char skin. Do not turn peppers, cook until skin blackens.

Remove from pan and wrap in clean towel to cool for 15-20 minutes. Using a paring knife, peel away skin, and cut peeled peppers into strips. Mix remaining oil and vinegar. Place peppers on serving dish and cover with dressing.

To serve, top with chopped garlic and green onions.

NUTRIONAL BREAKDOWN PER SERVING: Calories 70; Fat Grams 7; Carbohydrate Grams 3; Protein Grams 0; Cholesterol Grams 0; Sodium mg 1.

THE POINT SYSTEM: Calorie Points 1; Protein Points 0; Fat Grams 7; Sodium Points 0; Fiber Points 0; Carbohydrate Points 0; Cholesterol Points 0.

Leeks, Mushroom and Potato Soup

Serves: 12 – 1 cup servings
Preparation Time: 40 minutes
Equipment: French chef knife, cutting board, Kitchen Machine food cutter,
4-quart stockpot, blender

3	cups leeks rinsed well, sliced thin
2	cups fresh mushrooms, sliced blade #4 (to slice, place sideways in hopper)
4 ½	cups (1.1 L) water
4	cups red potatoes, diced
1	cup celery, sliced blade #4
1 ½	teaspoons, fresh or dry crushed tarragon
1	tablespoon fresh squeezed lemon juice
2	teaspoons low sodium Worcestershire sauce
½	teaspoon ground white pepper
3	tablespoons fresh chives or green onion, minced

Place 4-quart Stockpot (4 L) over medium heat until hot. Add leeks and mushrooms, cover, close the vent, and sweat down, about 10 minutes or until tender, stirring 2-3 times and replacing the cover.

Add water, potatoes, and celery. Bring to a simmer, cover, open vent, and cook until potatoes are tender, 25-30 minutes.

Place 1 cup vegetable mixture in blender to puree on low speed. Return puree to soup. Stir in tarragon, lemon juice, Worcestershire sauce, and white pepper.

To serve, ladle soup into individual bowls, sprinkle with chives or green onions.

NUTRIONAL BREAKDOWN PER SERVING: Calories 124; Fat Grams 0; Carbohydrate Grams 29; Protein Grams 4; Cholesterol Grams 0; Sodium mg 57.

THE POINT SYSTEM: Calorie Points 1½; Protein Points 0; Fat Grams 0; Sodium Points 2; Fiber Points 2; Carbohydrate Points 2; Cholesterol Points 0.

Indian Cauliflower Salad

Serves: 8
Preparation Time: 20 minutes
Equipment: Paring knife, cutting board, 11-inch mini WOK/saucier w/cover

1	head cauliflower
8	green onions
2	teaspoons black mustard seeds
2	teaspoons cumin seeds
2	teaspoons fennel seeds
½	teaspoon turmeric
½	cup (80 ml) warm water
¼	cup (60 ml) vegetable oil or sesame seed oil
½	cup fresh cilantro, chopped
1	head romaine lettuce, chopped or torn

Separate cauliflower into 1-inch (2.5 cm) florets, and set aside. With a paring knife, peel stems and cut stems into thin slices. Set aside. Stems can be sliced on the Kitchen Machine blade #4.

Trim onions and chop, including tops. Set aside.

Have spices and water ready right next to stove. Heat oil in WOK over medium-high heat; add mustard seeds, cumin seeds and fennel seeds. Reduce heat to low. Keep cover handy if seeds sputter and begin to pop. When seeds stop sputtering add turmeric and stir, add cauliflower and stir to coat. Add water, cover, open vent, and cook about 10 minutes.

To serve, place prepared romaine lettuce in salad bowl, top with green onions and cilantro, then add cauliflower and toss.

This dish is bright, attractive, unusual, and very good. Can be served with prepared brown rice or sliced sausage.

NUTRIONAL BREAKDOWN PER SERVING: Calories 93; Fat Grams 8; Carbohydrate Grams 5; Protein Grams 2; Cholesterol 0; Sodium mg 18.

THE POINT SYSTEM: Calorie Points 1; Protein Points 0; Fat Grams 8; Sodium Points 1; Fiber Points 0; Carbohydrate Points ½; Cholesterol Points 0.

Caesar Salad and Grilled Chicken

Serves: 4
Preparation Time: 20 minutes
Equipment: French chef knife, cutting board, kitchen machine, large skillet, large salad bowl

2	skinless, boneless chicken breasts
½	cup non-fat plain yogurt
I	teaspoon anchovy paste
I	teaspoon fresh lime juice
I	teaspoon balsamic vinegar
I	teaspoon Dijon mustard
½	teaspoon Worcestershire sauce (or low-sodium Worcestershire)
I	clove garlic, minced fine or pureed with a knife
¼	cup Parmesan cheese, freshly grated blade #1
I	head romaine lettuce cut into 1-inch (2.5 cm) wide strips
½	red onion, sliced very thin
½	red bell pepper, sliced into very thin rings

Preheat Large Skillet over medium heat. Sprinkle a few drops of water in the pan, if the water droplets 'dance', the pan is hot enough. Place chicken breasts in pan, cover, open the vent and brown, about 5 minutes. The chicken will release easily when seared sufficiently. Turn, cover and cook 3-5 minutes. Remove from the pan, cut into bite size pieces and place in the refrigerator to cool.

For salad dressing, blend together yogurt, anchovy paste, lime juice, balsamic vinegar, Dijon mustard, Worcestershire sauce, garlic, and Parmesan cheese. Place in refrigerator to cool.

To serve, in a large salad bowl add cut romaine, red onions, red pepper, chicken and dressing. Toss well, top with fresh cracked pepper.

NUTRIONAL BREAKDOWN PER SERVING: Calories 215; Fat Grams 6; Carbohydrate Grams 6; Protein Grams 33; Cholesterol mg 82; Sodium mg 382. (Sodium reduced by about ⅓ with low sodium Worcestershire sauce, see Nutritional Facts on label)

THE POINT SYSTEM: Calorie Points 3; Protein Points 4; Fat Grams 6; Sodium Points 16½; Fiber Points 0; Carbohydrate Points ½; Cholesterol Points 8.

Shrimp Dressing

Serves: 10 – Yields 2 cups
Preparation Time: 10 minutes (8 hours)
Equipment: French chef knife, cutting board, 2-quart stainless mixing bowl

1	cup low calorie mayonnaise
½	tube anchovy paste (1.6 ounce or 45 g)
1	cup low-fat yogurt
1	small can small shrimp, drained
1	small can mushroom pieces
1	clove garlic, minced fine or pureed with a knife
2	teaspoon onion, minced
1	tablespoon parsley, chopped

In a mixing bowl, combine all ingredients, cover and refrigerate about 8 hours for flavors to blend thoroughly.

To serve, spoon over lettuce and top with Homemade Croutons (page 70), or serve with steamed shrimp, lobster or crab.

NUTRIONAL BREAKDOWN PER SERVING: Calories 108; Fat Grams 7; Carbohydrate Grams 4; Protein Grams 7; Cholesterol mg 25; Sodium mg 182.

THE POINT SYSTEM: Calorie Points 1½; Protein Points 1; Fat Grams 7; Sodium Points 8; Fiber Points ½; Carbohydrate Points ½; Cholesterol Points 2½.

Patata-Piccata Salad

Serves: 6

Preparation Time: 2 hours

Equipment: French chef knife, cutting board, 3-quart saucepan, 3-quart stainless mixing bowl

I	pound (460 g) small red potatoes
I	cup (60 ml) Chablis or other dry wine
3	tablespoons chicken broth or homemade chicken stock
2	tablespoons water
I	tablespoon olive oil
2	teaspoons tarragon vinegar
2	teaspoons freshly squeezed lemon juice
¼	teaspoon sea salt or kosher salt (optional)
¼	teaspoon fresh ground black pepper
2	tablespoons raw sugar (optional, I tablespoon sugar)
3	tablespoons green onions, minced
3	tablespoons fresh parsley, minced
I	tablespoon capers, chopped

Scrub potatoes and remove blemishes. Place in 3-quart saucepan. Rinse and pour the excess water off. Place on medium-low heat with the cover on and vent closed. In 3-5 minutes the lid will spin freely on a cushion of moisture around the rim. This is the proper cooking temperature for waterless cooking. If the lid does not spin, increase the heat slightly. If the lid spits moisture, reduce the heat slightly. Cook until tender, about 30 minutes.

Allow the potatoes to cool slightly. With a knife, quarter potatoes and place in medium mixing bowl. Add wine; toss gently, and let stand about 15 minutes, tossing occasionally.

Combine chicken broth, water, olive oil, vinegar, lemon juice, salt, and pepper, and sugar, whisk and pour mixture over potatoes. Add green onions, parsley, and capers; toss gently. Cover and chill, about I hour before serving.

Nutritional breakdown includes 2 tablespoons sugar.

NUTRIONAL BREAKDOWN PER SERVING: Calories I I I; Fat Grams 2; Carbohydrate Grams 20; Protein Grams 2; Cholesterol mg 0; Sodium mg 172.

THE POINT SYSTEM: Calorie Points I ½; Protein Points 0; Fat Grams 2; Sodium Points 7½; Fiber Points I; Carbohydrate Points I ½; Cholesterol Points 0.

Green Beans and Fennel Salad

Serves: 8
Preparation Time: 45 minutes
Equipment: French chef knife, cutting board, Kitchen Machine food cutter,
4-quart stockpot, 2-quart steamer insert, small stainless mixing bowl

I	pound (460 g) fresh green beans, trimmed and cut 1-inch pieces
2	bulbs fresh fennel
½	pound (230 g) fresh mushrooms, cleaned, trimmed and quartered
2	tablespoons lemon zest, graded blade #1
I	cup (60 ml) balsamic vinegar
2	tablespoons water
2	tablespoons fresh squeezed lemon juice
2	tablespoons extra virgin olive oil
I	teaspoon raw sugar (optional)

Steam green beans over boiling water about 5 minutes with the cover on and the vent open.

Immediately, run under cold water or place green beans in ice bath to stop the cooking process. Drain, dry and place in large salad bowl.

Trim fennel leaves, reserve. Quarter bulb and remove core. Slice fennel bulb thinly, add to serving bowl along with quartered mushrooms, and sprinkle with lemon zest.

In a small mixing bowl combine vinegar, water, lemon juice, oil and sugar. Mix well, pour over salad and toss. Cover and refrigerate 30 minutes.

To serve, top with finely minced fennel leaves.

NUTRIONAL BREAKDOWN PER SERVING: Calories 68; Fat Grams 4; Carbohydrate Grams 10; Protein Grams 2; Cholesterol mg 0; Sodium mg 273.

THE POINT SYSTEM: Calorie Points 1; Protein Points 0; Fat Grams 4; Sodium Points 12; Fiber Points 0; Carbohydrate Points ½; Cholesterol Points 0.

Raita

Serves: 6
Preparation Time: 10 minutes
Equipment: French chef knife, cutting board, Kitchen Machine food cutter,
3-quart stainless mixing bowl

½ teaspoon sea salt or kosher salt (optional)
1 cup plain yogurt
1 clove garlic, minced
½ teaspoon freshly grated ginger blade #1
2 teaspoon white distilled vinegar
2 tablespoons mint leaves, chopped
¼ teaspoon black pepper, or to taste
¼ teaspoon of garam masala*
2 cucumbers with skin, sliced thin blade #4

*See recipe below for Garam Masala in the spice section, page 204.

In a mixing bowl, combine all ingredients except cucumbers. Just prior to serving add cucumber and mix well.

NOTE: The yogurt and cucumber mixture can take the fire out of hot spicy curry dishes. Serve as a small side salad.

NUTRIONAL BREAKDOWN PER SERVING: Calories 36; Fat Grams 0; Carbohydrate Grams 6; Protein Grams 3; Cholesterol mg 1; Sodium mg 143.

THE POINT SYSTEM: Calorie Points ½; Protein Points 0; Fat Grams 0; Sodium Points 6; Fiber Points 0; Carbohydrate Points ½; Cholesterol Points 0.

Company Tossed Salad

Serves: 8
Preparation Time: 15 minutes
Equipment: French chef knife, cutting board, Kitchen Machine food cutter, 8-inch Chef Pan

1	large head green leaf or romaine lettuce
3	strips bacon, sliced ¼-inch (0.5 cm) (optional, Canadian bacon)
2	cloves garlic, minced
¼	cup (60 ml) red wine vinegar dressing
5	mushrooms, sliced blade #4 (to slice, place sideways in hopper)
	Homemade croutons (recipe below)

Clean and dry greens in salad spinner or on paper towels, refrigerate covered. Tear or cut greens prior to mixing with other ingredients.

In the 8-inch chef pan, over medium high heat, cook bacon about 5 minutes, add garlic, sauté 3-4 4 minutes and remove with slotted spoon to drain on paper towels. Set skillet with drippings aside.

Just prior to serving, heat bacon drippings, deglaze pan with prepared dressing. Pour over mixed greens and mushrooms, toss well.

To serve, divide between individual salad plates and top with bacon bits and homemade croutons.

NUTRIONAL BREAKDOWN PER SERVING: Calories 94; Fat Grams 5; Carbohydrate Grams 10; Protein Grams ½; Cholesterol mg 5; Sodium mg 180.

THE POINT SYSTEM: Calorie Points 0; Protein Points 4; Fat Grams 5; Sodium Points 8; Fiber Points 0; Carbohydrate Points ½; Cholesterol Points ½.

Homemade Croutons

Serves: 8
Preparation Time: 10 minutes

2	tablespoons of low calorie margarine or unsalted butter
1	tablespoon basil
1	teaspoon parsley flakes
½	teaspoon ground black pepper
4	slices toasted bread, cubed
2	tablespoons grated Parmesan cheese, blade #1

Melt margarine or butter in small skillet. Add basil, parsley, and pepper. Place cubed bread in stainless mixing bowl with Parmesan cheese. Drizzle butter mixture over bread, cover and shake to coat.

Italian Salad Dressing

Serves: 12 / 1-ounce servings
Preparation Time: 5 minutes
Equipment: French chef knife, cutting board, kitchen Machine food cutter

5	clove garlic, minced or pureed with French chef knife
¼	cup (180 ml) olive oil
½	cup balsamic vinegar
⅓	cup (80 ml) red wine
2	teaspoons raw sugar (optional, 1 teaspoon)
½	teaspoon salt (optional)
1	teaspoon pepper
1	tablespoon sweet basil (fresh or dried)
1	tablespoon fresh parsley, minced

In a covered salad jar, combine Italian all ingredients. Shake to blend and serve over salad greens.

Nutritional breakdown includes sugar and salt as listed in the ingredients.

NUTRIONAL BREAKDOWN PER SERVING: Calories 131; Fat Grams 14; Carbohydrate Grams 2; Protein Grams 0; Cholesterol mg 0; Sodium mg 94.

THE POINT SYSTEM: Calorie Points 1½; Protein Points 0; Fat Grams 14; Sodium Points 4; Fiber Points 0; Carbohydrate Points 0; Cholesterol Points 0.

Variation, add 1 small can sliced olives, drained, and ¼ cup Parmesan cheese, grated blade #1.

French Salad Dressing

Yields: 15 / 3-ounce servings
Preparation Time: 10 minutes
Equipment: French chef knife, cutting board, Kitchen Machine food cutter

1	10 ¾ ounce (305 g) can tomato soup
⅓	cup (80 ml) vinegar, white distiller or red wine vinegar
¼	cup (60 ml) water
1	cup raw sugar (or ¼ cup sugar substitute, check package for quantity relationship)
1	cup (240 ml) light olive oil, sesame seed oil, or vegetable oil
½	tablespoon paprika
4	cloves garlic, minced fine
½	teaspoon salt (optional)

Combine ingredients in a large covered jar, and xix or shake to blend. Shake before each use.

Nutritional breakdown includes sugar as listed in ingredients above.

NUTRIONAL BREAKDOWN PER SERVING: Calories 198; Fat Grams 15; Carbohydrate Grams 17; Protein Grams 0; Cholesterol mg 0; Sodium mg 374.

THE POINT SYSTEM: Calorie Points 2½; Protein Points 0; Fat Grams 15; Sodium Points 16; Fiber Points 0; Carbohydrate Points 1; Cholesterol Points 0.

Southwest Vinegar Dressing

Yields: 10 cups
Serves: 40
Preparation Time: 10 minutes (fermentation time 2 weeks)
Equipment: French chef knife, cutting board, 3-quart saucepan

1	large bunch fresh cilantro
12	fresh jalapeno peppers, seeded, cut in half lengthwise
12	cloves garlic, peeled and cut in half lengthwise
1	lime, sliced thin
12	dried tomato halves
1	teaspoon black peppercorns
5	17-ounce (2.5 L) bottles white wine vinegar
	Additional fresh cilantro sprigs and lime slices (optional)

Twist cilantro stems gently. Place cilantro, jalapeno, garlic, lime, tomatoes, and peppercorns in a large glass container or Mason jar, with lid.

In the 3-quart saucepan (3 L), bring vinegar to a simmer. Remove from heat, and let stand, about 5 minutes. Pour hot vinegar over cilantro mixture. Cover and let stand at room temperature 2 weeks.

Pour mixture through a large wire-mesh strainer into decorative bottles, discarding solids. Thread additional cilantro sprigs and lime slices on a wooden skewer, if desired, and place in bottle. Seal and store in a cool dark place.

NUTRIONAL BREAKDOWN PER SERVING: Calories 10; Fat Grams 0; Carbohydrate Grams 2; Protein Grams 1; Cholesterol mg 0; Sodium mg 110.

THE POINT SYSTEM: Calorie Points 0; Protein Points 0; Fat Grams 0; Sodium Points 5; Fiber Points 0; Carbohydrate Points 0; Cholesterol Points 0.

Tomato Herb Dressing

Yields: 11 cups
Serves: 40
Preparation Time: 10 minutes (fermentation time 2 weeks)
Equipment: French chef knife, cutting board, 4-quart stockpot

10	large sprigs fresh rosemary
6	large sprigs fresh basil
4	large sprigs fresh oregano
12	cloves garlic, peeled and halved
10	dried tomato halves
1	teaspoon black peppercorns
3	32-ounce (1 L) bottles red wine vinegar
	Additional rosemary (optional)

Twist stems of herbs gently, and crush garlic with back of spoon or side of knife. Place herbs and garlic in a large glass container or Mason jar, with lid. Add tomatoes and peppercorns. Set aside.

In the 4-quart Stockpot (4 L), bring vinegar to a simmer, remove from heat and let stand, about 5 minutes. Pour warm vinegar over herb mixture. Cover and let stand at room temperature 2 weeks.

Pour vinegar mixture through a large wire mesh strainer into decorative bottles, discarding solids. Add additional rosemary, if desired. Seal and store bottles and store in a cool, dry place.

NUTRIONAL BREAKDOWN PER SERVING: Calories 17; Fat Grams 0; Carbohydrate Grams 5; Protein Grams 0; Cholesterol mg 0; Sodium mg 3.

THE POINT SYSTEM: Calorie Points 0; Protein Points 0; Fat Grams 0; Sodium Points 0; Fiber Points 0; Carbohydrate Points 0; Cholesterol Points 0.

Apricot Apple Chutney

Excellent complement when serving pork, lamb, chicken and when served
on toasted French bread.
Serves: 20
Preparation Time: 1 hour
Equipment: French chef knife, cutting board, Kitchen Machine food cutter, 2-quart saucepan

1½	pounds (690 g) green apples chopped and peeled blade #3
6	dried apricots, sliced thin
¼	cup (180 ml) water
1¼	cups brown sugar, or raw sugar
¼	cup raisins
1	onion, chopped and peeled blade #3
1	clove garlic, minced
½	cup (160 ml) apple cider vinegar
1	cinnamon stick
4	cloves
1	bay leaf
½	teaspoon garam masala*
1	teaspoon sea salt or kosher salt
½	teaspoon cayenne pepper

Cut apples in half and remove the stem with a paring knife and the core with a teaspoon. Using the Kitchen Machine and blade #3, place the skin-side up away from the blade, chop and peel apples.

Bring water to a simmer in 2-quart saucepan (2 L) stir in sugar and add remaining ingredients. Cover open vent and simmer 40 minutes. With a spoon, remove cinnamon stick, cloves and bay leaf.

See *Garam Masala recipe on page 204.

NUTRITIONAL BREAKDOWN PER SERVING: Calories 108; Fat Grams 0; Carbohydrate Grams 27; Protein Grams 0; Cholesterol mg 0; Sodium mg 115.

THE POINT SYSTEM: Calorie Points 1 ½; Protein Points 0; Fat Grams 0; Sodium Points 5; Fiber Points 1; Carbohydrate Points 2; Cholesterol Points 0.

Stuffed Mushrooms

Serves: 12
Preparation Time: 20 minutes
Equipment: French chef knife, cutting board, Kitchen Machine food cutter,
3-quart stainless mixing bowl, large skillet

2	cloves, garlic minced or pureed with a knife
¼	cup onions, minced
I	tablespoon fresh parsley, chopped
½	cup Velveeta Italian cheese, shredded blade #3
I	6-ounce (170 g) can crab meat, drained (or freshly boiled)
I2	large mushroom caps, stems removed
½	teaspoon paprika

NOTE: Soft cheese shreds easier when firmed by placing in freezer for 15-30 minutes.

In a mixing bowl, combine garlic, onions, parsley, cheese, and crab meat, mix well, and fill each mushroom cap with mixture.

Place stuffed mushrooms in large, skillet, cover, close the vent and cook waterless until Vapor Seal is formed (approximately 5 minutes). Reduce heat to low for an additional 10 minutes.

To serve, remove from skillet with slotted spoon to serving plate and sprinkle with paprika.

NUTRITIONAL BREAKDOWN PER SERVING: Calories 43; Fat Grams 3; Carbohydrate Grams 2; Protein Grams 4; Cholesterol mg 15; Sodium mg 160.

THE POINT SYSTEM: Calorie Points ½; Protein Points ½; Fat Grams 3; Sodium Points 7; Fiber Points 0; Carbohydrate Points 0; Cholesterol Points I ½.

Hot Crab Dip

Serves: 15
Preparation Time: 15 minutes
Equipment: French chef knife, cutting board, Kitchen Machine food cutter,
5-quart electric saucepan

½	cup Parmesan cheese, grated blade #1
2	cups fat free or low fat mayonnaise
1	6 ounce (170 g) can Dungeness crab meat
1	13 ounce (370 g) jar artichoke hearts, drained and chopped
	Tortilla chips
1	green onion, chopped
½	teaspoon cayenne pepper

In the 5-quart electric saucepan, combine Parmesan cheese, mayonnaise, crab and artichokes. Set heat control at simmer, about 15 minutes.

To serve, ladle crab mixture into serving bowl, top with green onions and sprinkle with cayenne pepper. Serve with tortilla chips.

NUTRITIONAL BREAKDOWN PER SERVING: Calories 59; Fat Grams 1; Carbohydrate Grams 9; Protein Grams 4; Cholesterol mg 13; Sodium mg 527.

THE POINT SYSTEM: Calorie Points 1; Protein Points 0; Fat Grams 1; Sodium Points 23; Fiber Points 0; Carbohydrate Points ½; Cholesterol Points 1.

Wrapped Chestnuts

Serves: 12
Preparation Time: 30 minutes
Equipment: 13-inch chef pan or 12-inch electric skillet, 3-quart stainless mixing bowl

24	strips bacon, cut in half or Canadian bacon or prosciutto
1	can water chestnuts, drained
1	cup (240 ml) reduced calorie ketchup
1	cup (240 ml) honey
24	toothpicks
2	tablespoons fresh parsley, chopped

Wrap one-half slice bacon around one whole water chestnut, secure with toothpick.

Preheat skillet over medium heat (350°F/180°C for electric skillet). Place bacon wrapped water chestnuts in pan, cover, open vent and brown until crisp, about 5-7 minutes. Turn chestnuts and repeat the process until bacon is cooked to desired crispness on all sides. When finished cooking, drain grease from pan, reduce heat to low (simmer for Electric Skillet).

In a mixing bowl, while chestnuts are cooking, combine ketchup and honey. After grease has been removed from skillet, pour mixture over wrapped chestnuts. Cover; continue cooking on low heat about 10 minutes, turn occasionally to glaze.

To serve, remove to large serving platter, top with parsley and garnish with orange slices.

NUTRITIONAL BREAKDOWN PER SERVING: Calories 227; Fat Grams 6; Carbohydrate Grams 38; Protein Grams 6; Cholesterol mg 11; Sodium mg 210.

THE POINT SYSTEM: Calorie Points 3; Protein Points 1; Fat Grams 6; Sodium Points 9; Fiber Points 0; Carbohydrate Points 2½; Cholesterol Points 1.

Sesame Chicken Wings

Serves: 6
Preparation Time: 25 minutes
Equipment: French chef knife, cutting board, Kitchen Machine food cutter,
2-quart stainless mixing bowl, 11-inch mini WOK

12	chicken wings
1	tablespoon precooked black beans
1	tablespoon water
2	cloves garlic, minced
1	tablespoon fresh ginger, grated blade #1
3	tablespoons dry sherry or rice wine
¼	teaspoon black pepper
1	tablespoon sesame seeds
1	green onion, chopped

Using a knife or poultry shears, trim and discard wing tips, separate wings into two parts.

In mixing bowl, crush beans with fork, add water and set aside.

To cook, preheat WOK on medium-high heat; add chicken, garlic, and ginger. Stir fry until wings are lightly browned. Add soy sauce and sherry, stir fry 1-2 minutes. Add soaked black beans, pepper and sesame seeds. Cover with vent open; reduce heat to low, simmer 8-10 minutes.

Uncover, increase heat to medium-high. To glaze wings in sauce, stir occasionally until liquid has almost evaporated and wings are glazed in sauce. Remove from heat, sprinkle with sesame seeds, and stir to coat.

To serve, arrange wings on serving platter, top with chopped green onions and garnish with sliced lemon, lime or orange.

Variation, to reduce cholesterol and fat calories, trim or remove skin from chicken.

NUTRITIONAL BREAKDOWN PER SERVING: Calories 173; Fat Grams 11; Carbohydrate Grams 2; Protein Grams 14; Cholesterol mg 44; Sodium mg 269.

THE POINT SYSTEM: Calorie Points 2 ½; Protein Points 2; Fat Grams 11; Sodium Points 12; Fiber Points 0; Carbohydrate Points 0; Cholesterol Points 4.

Hummus

Serves: 8 – Yields 4 cups
Preparation Time: 10 minutes
Equipment: French chef knife, cutting board, electric food processor or blender

2	cups chickpeas, cooked or canned
¼	cup (60 ml) freshly squeezed lemon juice
½	cup (120 ml) water
3	tablespoons vegetable oil or sesame seed oil
2	cloves garlic, minced fine
½	teaspoon sea salt or kosher salt (optional)
1	cup Tahini*

In a food processor, puree chickpeas with lemon juice; add water as needed to keep blending. Add remaining ingredients, puree to a creamy paste.

To serve, Hummus may be served in many ways and with a variety of garnishes. For a luncheon salad plate, arrange humus on lettuce leaves, sprinkle with paprika, and garnish with sliced cucumbers, cherry tomatoes, carrot slices, and serve with whole wheat bread, wheat crackers or Nan Bread**.

For a sandwich spread, cut pieces of Middle Eastern Flatbread** (pita) in half and fill pockets with humus. Add garnishes such as shredded lettuce, chopped tomatoes, chopped cucumbers, etc. Or spread on cracker or toast.

For a dip, serve with fresh cut vegetables.

Tahini*, see recipe on page 205.

Middle Eastern Flat Bread** recipe on page 167

NUTRITIONAL BREAKDOWN PER SERVING: Calories 211; Fat Grams 16; Carbohydrate Grams 14; Protein Grams 6; Cholesterol mg 2; Sodium mg 264.

THE POINT SYSTEM: Calorie Points 3; Protein Points 1; Fat Grams 16; Sodium Points 11; Fiber Points 1 ½; Carbohydrate Points 1; Cholesterol Points 0.

Beef, Lamb & Pork...

Boeuf Bourguinon

Beef Stew
Serves: 8
Preparation Time: 2½ hours
Equipment: French chef knife, cutting board, 6-quart stockpot, medium skillet

2	pounds (1 kg) sirloin steak cut in ¼-inch cubes
3	shallots, peeled and chopped
3	cloves garlic, chopped
4	tablespoons flour
3	cups (720 ml) dry red wine
1	bay leaf
2	cups (480 ml) beef stock, heated
1	teaspoon basil
1	teaspoon fresh parsley, chopped
2	tablespoons unsalted butter
24	pearl onions, peeled
1	pound (460 g) fresh mushrooms, cleaned and halved
	parsley leaves for garnish

Preheat 6-quart (6 L) Stockpot over medium heat. Add sirloin and sear on all sides. Add shallots and garlic, sauté for about 5 minutes. Sprinkle flour over meat a tablespoon at a time, stirring to combine ingredients, sauté 4-5 minutes.

Add wine to deglaze pan. Add bay leaf and bring to a simmer over medium-high heat. Cook uncovered until liquid is reduced by about two-thirds. Add beef stock, basil, and parsley. Cover, open vent, reduce heat to low and simmer 2 hours.

About 30 minutes before serving, heat butter in skillet over medium heat. Add pearl onions and mushrooms, sauté about 5 minutes, and then add to stew.

To serve, ladle into individual serving bowl, top with parsley leaves, and serve with toasted Italian or French garlic bread (see recipe, page 179).

NUTRITIONAL BREAKDOWN PER SERVING: Calories 345; Fat Grams 6; Carbohydrate Grams 14; Protein Grams 50; Cholesterol mg 50; Sodium mg 847 (508 with homemade beef stock).

THE POINT SYSTEM: Calorie Points 4 ½; Protein Points 6; Fat Grams 6; Sodium Points 37 (22 with homemade beef stock); Fiber Points 1; Carbohydrate Points 1; Cholesterol Points 5.

Saucy Beef and Noodles

Serves: 6

Preparation Time: 1 hour

Equipment: French chef knife, cutting board, Kitchen Machine food cutter, 10-inch chef pan

1	pound (460 g) lean round steak, trimmed and sliced ½ inch (1.5 cm) thick
2	cups fresh mushrooms, sliced blade #4 (to slice, lay sideways in hopper)
½	cup, celery chopped
3	green onions, chopped
1	clove garlic, chopped
2	8 ounce (230 g) cans tomato sauce, no salt added
	or 1½ pounds plum tomatoes, peeled, seeded and chopped
½	cup (80 ml) Chablis or other dry white wine
1	tablespoon fresh squeezed lemon juice
1	bay leaf
½	teaspoon dried oregano
¼	teaspoon dried rosemary, crushed
¼	teaspoon ground pepper
3	cups hot, cooked, unsalted medium egg noodles.

Preheat 10-inch chef pan over medium-high heat. Add steak and brown on both sides. Remove steak to platter. Reduce heat to medium-low; add mushrooms, celery, green onions, and garlic. Sauté until vegetables are tender. Add steak and tomato sauce, and next 6 ingredients. Cover, close vent, reduce the heat to low, and simmer 45 minutes or until meat is tender. Remove and discard the bay leaf. Serve over hot cooked egg noodles.

NUTRITIONAL BREAKDOWN PER SERVING: Calories 309; Fat Grams 12; Carbohydrate Grams 29; Protein Grams 19; Cholesterol mg 73; Sodium mg 560.

THE POINT SYSTEM: Calorie Points 4; Protein Points 2; Fat Grams 12; Sodium Points 3; Fiber Points 2; Carbohydrate Points 2; Cholesterol Points 7.

Beef with Broccoli

Serves: 6

Preparation Time: 1 hour 15 minutes

Equipment: 3-quart saucepan, French chef knife, cutting board, Kitchen Machine food cutter, 3-quart stainless mixing bowl, paring knife, 1-quart stainless mixing bowl, 13-inch chef pan

3	cups cooked rice
1	pound (460 g) lean round steak
1	tablespoon dry sherry, divided
2	teaspoons cornstarch
1	tablespoon cornstarch
2	teaspoons raw sugar, divided (sugar may be reduced to two ½ teaspoons)
2	teaspoons sesame oil
2	teaspoons reduce-sodium soy sauce, divided
1	pound (460 g) fresh broccoli
½	cup (120 ml) chicken broth or homemade chicken stock
1	tablespoon hoisin sauce
½	teaspoon ground white pepper
1	tablespoon safflower oil
1	tablespoon ginger, freshly grated blade #1
2	teaspoons garlic, minced
1	medium sweet red pepper cut it julienne strips
1	tablespoon sesame seeds, toasted

In large mixing bowl, combine 1 tablespoon dry sherry, 2 teaspoons cornstarch, 1 teaspoon sugar, 1 teaspoon sesame oil, 1 teaspoon soy sauce, stir well. Add steak, tossing gently; cover and marinate in refrigerate 1 hour.

With a paring knife, trim broccoli and remove tough ends of lower stalks. Cut off florets, set aside. Slice stalks in ¼-inch (75 mm) strips, set aside.

In small mixing bowl, combine 1 tablespoon cornstarch and 1 tablespoon dry sherry, stir well. Add chicken stock, hoisin sauce, 1 teaspoon sugar, 1 teaspoon sesame oil, 1 teaspoon soy sauce, and white pepper; stir well and set aside.

Preheat skillet over medium-high heat, add safflower oil; allow to heat 1 minute. Add ginger and garlic, stir fry about 20-30 seconds. Add beef and marinade, stir fry 1 minute. Add broccoli and red peppers, stir fry 2-3 minutes to desired doneness. Add cornstarch mixture and continue to stir. Reduce heat to low, cover with vent closed, and cook 2 minutes or until mixture slightly thickens. To Serve: Spoon beef with broccoli over rice.

NUTRITIONAL BREAKDOWN PER SERVING: Calories 343; Fat Grams 9; Carbohydrate Grams 36; Protein Grams 31; Cholesterol mg 64; Sodium mg 348 (209 with homemade Chicken Stock).

THE POINT SYSTEM: Calorie Points 4 ½; Protein Points 4; Fat Grams 9; Sodium Points 15; Fiber Points 2 ½; Carbohydrate Points 2 ½; Cholesterol Points 6.

Griddle Kabobs

Serves: 8
Preparation Time: 55 minutes
Equipment: 3-quart saucepan, French chef knife, cutting board, 2-burner breakfast griddle

8	wooden skewers
2	pounds (1 kg) rump roast, cut into 2-inch cubes
I	8 ounce (230 g) reduced calorie Italian Dressing or homemade*
8	pearl onions, peeled
8	cherry tomatoes
I	small zucchini squash, cut in I-inch (2.5 cm) cubes
8	whole mushrooms
I	green pepper cut in I-inch (2.5 cm) pieces

Using poultry shears, trim blunt end of skewers to width of griddle.

Marinade beef cubes in Italian dressing, 30 minutes to I hour.

While beef is marinating prepare rice or sweet potatoes as side dish to Kabobs.

Skewer beef cubes and vegetables.

Preheat griddle over two burners on medium-high heat. Sprinkle a few drops of water on the griddle. If the water droplets evaporate the pan is not hot enough, when water droplets dance, the skillet has reached the proper cooking temperature for grilling on top of the range.

Place Kabobs carefully on hot griddle. They will immediately stick to the skillet until seared sufficiently (about 4-5 minutes per side. When Kabobs loosen easily, turn and repeat the process until all four sides are cooked.

To Serve: Baste with remaining marinade, if desired. Sprinkle with fresh ground pepper. Serve immediately over rice or with sweet potatoes cooked the waterless way.

Homemade Italian Salad Dressing* see page 71.

NUTRITIONAL BREAKDOWN PER SERVING: Calories 250; Fat Grams 9; Carbohydrate Grams 19; Protein Grams 25; Cholesterol mg 67; Sodium mg 309.

THE POINT SYSTEM: Calorie Points 3½; Protein Points 3; Fat Grams 9; Sodium Points 13; Fiber Points 2; Carbohydrate Points 1; Cholesterol Points 7.

Beef and Chinese Vegetables

Serves: 4
Preparation Time: 20 minutes
Equipment: French chef knife, cutting board, Kitchen Machine food cutter, 3-quart saucepan,
11-inch Mini-WOK/saucier, 1-quart stainless mixing bowl

1	pound (460 g) lean beef round steak sliced across the grain ¼ inch strips
⅔	cup green beans, trimmed and sliced ¼ inch pieces
2	carrots, sliced blade #4 or waffle cut blade #5, about ⅔ cup
2	small turnips, julienned blade #3, about ⅔ cup
4	cauliflower florets, sliced with French chefs knife, about ⅔ cup
¼	head Chinese cabbage, shredded #5 blade, about ⅔ cup
½	teaspoon fresh ginger, grated #1 blade
⅛	teaspoon garlic powder
1	tablespoon low sodium soy sauce
⅔	cup (160 ml) water
4	green onions, chopped

Place all the vegetables in the 3-quart saucepan, rinse with cold water and pour the water off. The water that clings to the vegetables is sufficient for cooking the waterless way. Cover the pan, close the vent and cook over medium-low heat. When the cover spins freely on a cushion of water, the vapor seal is formed, 3 to 5 minutes. After forming the vapor seal, cook about 10 minutes. Vegetables should be tender but crisp.

In mixing bowl, combine cornstarch, ginger, garlic powder, soy sauce, and water, mix well, set aside.

When vegetables are almost done, preheat WOK over medium-high heat. When hot, add beef and stir-fry about 3-5 minutes. Add cornstarch mixture, simmer, and cook until mixture thickens.

To serve, place vegetables on individual serving plates, spoon over beef mixture, and top with green onions.

NUTRITIONAL BREAKDOWN PER SERVING: Calories 202; Fat Grams 5; Carbohydrate Grams 12; Protein Grams 27; Cholesterol mg 50; Sodium mg 243.

THE POINT SYSTEM: Calorie Points 2½; Protein Points 3; Fat Grams 5; Sodium Points 10½; Fiber Points 1; Carbohydrate Points 1; Cholesterol Points 5.

Sauerkraut and Pork Skillet

Serves: 4
Preparation Time: 45 minutes
Equipment: French chef knife, cutting board, large skillet

4	pork chops, trimmed of fat
1	medium onion, sliced and separated into rings
1	clove garlic, minced
1	16 ounce (460 g) can, sauerkraut drained
½	cup (120 ml) apple juice
1	teaspoon caraway seeds
¼	teaspoon thyme
¼	teaspoon pepper
1	apple, cored and sliced

Preheat skillet over medium-high heat for 3-4 minutes. Sprinkle a few drops of water in the pan. If the water droplets dance, the pan is ready. If the water evaporates, the pan is not hot enough. Place the pork chops in the hot, dry skillet, which will be about 400°F (200°C). Cover the pan, open vent, cook pork chops until they release easily from the skillet, 4 to 5 minutes. Turn, cover and brown on other side, 4 to 5 minutes. Remove pork chops from pan and set aside.

To the skillet, add onion rings and garlic. Cover, close the vent, and reduce to low-heat. Cook about 5 minutes. Add sauerkraut, apple juice, caraway seeds, thyme and pepper. Stir to blend. Place pork chops on top; cover and simmer 10 minutes. Add apple slices; cover and simmer 5 minutes.

To serve, place pork chops to individual plates, surround with sauerkraut mixture, top with cooked apples, and garnish with fresh apple slices.

NUTRITIONAL BREAKDOWN PER SERVING: Calories 214; Fat Grams 9; Carbohydrate Grams 16; Protein Grams 17; Cholesterol mg 53; Sodium mg 1170.

THE POINT SYSTEM: Calorie Points 3; Protein Points 2; Fat Grams 9; Sodium Points 51; Fiber Points 1; Carbohydrate Points 1; Cholesterol Points 5.

Swedish Meatballs

Serves: 4
Preparation Time: 30 minutes
Equipment: French chef knife, cutting board, 3-quart stainless mixing bowl,
large skillet, 2-quart stainless mixing bowl

1	pound (460 g) ground chuck*
1	egg or 2 egg whites
1	teaspoon garlic powder
½	teaspoon fresh basil, chopped (or dried)
¼	teaspoon oregano
¼	teaspoon fresh parsley, chopped (or dried)
2	tablespoons tomato paste
½	cup (120 ml) ketchup
¼	cup (60 ml) ginger ale
1	8 ounce (230 g) can evaporated milk
1	cup (240 ml) beef broth or homemade beef stock

In large mixing bowl, combine ground chuck, egg, garlic powder, basil, oregano and parsley. Mix thoroughly, and form into 1-inch (2.5 cm) size meatballs.

Preheat skillet over medium-high heat for 3-4 minutes. Sprinkle a few drops of water in the pan. If the water droplets dance, the pan is ready. If the water evaporates, the pan is not hot enough. Place the meatballs in the hot, dry pan, which will be about 400°F (200°C). Cover the pan, open the vent, and brown until meatballs release easily from the skillet, 4 to 5 minutes. Turn meatballs, cover pan, and repeat the process until meatballs are browned on all sides, about 3-4 minutes each side.

While the meatballs are browning, in the 2-quart mixing bowl, combine tomato paste, ketchup, ginger ale, evaporated milk and beef stock. When meatballs are browned on all sides, remove excess grease from skillet, and pour beef stock mixture into the skillet. Reduce heat to low, cover, close vent, and simmer 10 minutes.

*Ground Turkey, chicken, pork or veal (or a combination thereof) can be substituted for ground chuck.

To serve, spoon Swedish Meatballs and sauce over egg noodles or rice, or serve as appetizer.

NUTRITIONAL BREAKDOWN PER SERVING: Calories 266; Fat Grams 9; Carbohydrate Grams 11; Protein Grams 36; Cholesterol mg 36; Sodium mg 828 (503 with homemade beef stock).

THE POINT SYSTEM: Calorie Points 3½; Protein Points 4½; Fat Grams 9; Sodium Points 36 (22 with homemade beef stock); Fiber Points 0; Carbohydrate Points ½; Cholesterol Points 4.

Meatballs á la Swiss

Serves: 4
Preparation Time: 30 minutes
Equipment: French chef knife, cutting board, Kitchen Machine food cutter, 3-quart stainless mixing bowl, large skillet, 2-quart stainless mixing bowl

1	pound (460 g) ground lean beef
⅔	cup (160 ml) evaporated milk, divided
¼	cup (60 ml) ketchup
1	tablespoon fresh parsley, chopped (or dried)
1	tablespoon Dijon mustard
1	teaspoon black pepper
1	10 ½ ounce (300 g) can cream of chicken soup or Sauce Supreme
½	cup Swiss cheese, shredded blade #3
3	drops Crystal hot sauce, or Tabasco

In a large mixing bowl, combine beef, ½ cup evaporated milk, ketchup, parsley, mustard, and pepper. Shape into 16 meatballs, about 1½-inch (4 cm) in diameter.

Preheat skillet over medium-high heat for 3-4 minutes. Sprinkle a few drops of water in the pan. If the water droplets dance, the pan is ready. If the water evaporates, the pan is not hot enough. Place the meatballs in the hot, dry pan, which will be about 400°F (200°C). Cover the pan, open the vent, and brown meatballs until they release easily from the skillet, 4 to 5 minutes. Repeat the process until meatballs are browned on all sides.

While the meatballs are browning, in the 2-quart mixing bowl, combine soup, cheese, ⅓ cup evaporated milk, water, and hot sauce. Drain excess grease from skillet, to deglaze skillet add soup mixture to meatballs. Reduce the heat to low, cover, close vent, and simmer 15 minutes.

To serve, spoon meatballs and sauce over egg noodles or rice, or serve as and appetizer.

NUTRITIONAL BREAKDOWN PER SERVING: Calories 302; Fat Grams 18; Carbohydrate Grams 11; Protein Grams 22; Cholesterol mg 70; Sodium mg 650 (390 mg with homemade Sauce Supreme).

THE POINT SYSTEM: Calorie Points 4; Protein Points 3; Fat Grams 18; Sodium Points 28 (17 points with homemade Sauce Supreme); Fiber Points 0; Carbohydrate Points ½; Cholesterol Points 7.

Italian Meatballs

Yields: 20 meatballs
Preparation Time: 1 hour
Equipment: French chef knife, cutting board, Kitchen Machine food cutter, 6-quart stockpot,
large stainless mixing bowl, large skillet

SAUCE

1	tablespoon olive oil
½	onion, peeled and chopped blade #3
½	cup green pepper, chopped
2	cloves garlic, minced
2	16 ounce (460 g) cans whole tomatoes,
	or 1½ pounds plum tomatoes, peeled, seeded and chopped
1	cup (240 ml) tomato puree
1	teaspoon raw sugar
½	teaspoon oregano, dried or fresh chopped
½	pound (230 g) mushrooms, sliced blade #4 (to slice, lay sideways in hopper)

MEATBALLS

1	pound (460 g) lean ground beef
½	pound (230 g) ground pork or veal
1	cup Parmesan cheese, grated blade #1
1	egg or 2 egg whites
½	cup Italian bread crumbs
½	cup fresh parsley, chopped
3	cloves garlic, minced

For sauce, preheat 6-quart stockpot over medium heat for 3-4 minutes. Add olive oil, sauté onions, green pepper and garlic until softened. Add all remaining ingredients, mix well, reduce the heat to low, cover, open vent, and simmer for 1 hour. Stir occasionally.

For meatballs, in large mixing bowl, combine meat, cheese, egg, bread crumbs, parsley, and garlic. Mix thoroughly, and form into twenty 1½-inch (2.5 cm) size meatballs. Preheat skillet over medium-high heat for 3-4 minutes. Place the meatballs in the hot, dry pan, cover, open vent, brown until meatballs release easily from the skillet, 4 to 5 minutes. Turn and repeat the process until meatballs are browned on all sides. Remove from pan to sauce. Remove excess grease from skillet, deglaze skillet with 1-2 cup of sauce, simmer for 5 minutes, and add to sauce. Stir.

To serve, spoon Italian Meatballs and sauce over pasta or serve with risotto, or serve on Italian bread for meatball sandwich.

NUTRITIONAL BREAKDOWN PER SERVING: Calories 280; Fat Grams 13; Carbohydrate Grams 19; Protein Grams 21; Cholesterol mg 52; Sodium mg 473 (284 with fresh plum tomatoes).

THE POINT SYSTEM: Calorie Points 3½; Protein Points 3; Fat Grams 13; Sodium Points 20½ (13 with fresh plum tomatoes); Fiber Points 1; Carbohydrate Points 1½; Cholesterol Points 5.

Ground Beef Skillet Casserole

Serves: 6
Preparation Time: 1 hour
Equipment: French chef knife, cutting board, Kitchen Machine food cutter, large skillet

½	pound (230 g) lean ground beef
1	green pepper, chopped fine
1	onion, peeled, halved and chopped blade #3
1	cup celery, diced
¼	teaspoon low-sodium Worcestershire sauce
¼	teaspoon pepper
1 ½	cups low-sodium tomato juice or V8
1	cup macaroni, uncooked
½	cup mushrooms, sliced blade #4 (to slice, lay sideways in hopper)

Preheat skillet over medium-high heat for 3-4 minutes. Sprinkle a few drops of water in the pan. If the water droplets dance, the pan is ready. If the water evaporates, the pan is not hot enough. Place the ground beef in the hot, dry pan, which will be about 400°F (200°C). Cover the pan, and open the vent and dry sauté until cooked, about 10 minutes, stir occasionally.

Drain excess grease from skillet, and add green pepper, onions and celery. Reduce the heat to medium, cover with vent open, and cook 10 minutes.

Add remaining ingredients, reduce the heat to low, cover with the vent closed, and simmer 40-45 minutes.

To serve, spoon into individual serving bowls, top with fresh chopped cilantro or parsley.

NUTRITIONAL BREAKDOWN PER SERVING: Calories 139; Fat Grams 5; Carbohydrate Grams 15; Protein Grams 9; Cholesterol mg 23; Sodium mg 238.

THE POINT SYSTEM: Calorie Points 2; Protein Points 1; Fat Grams 5; Sodium Points 10; Fiber Points 1; Carbohydrate Points 1; Cholesterol Points 2.

Pork 'n Pineapple Chili

Serves: 12
Preparation Time: 3 hours
Equipment: French chef knife, cutting board, Kitchen Machine food cutter, 6-quart stockpot

2	pounds (920 g) lean pork cut into 1-inch (2.5 cm) cubes
3	cloves garlic, minced
2	medium onions, halved, peeled and chopped blade #3
1	28 ounce (800 g) can chopped tomatoes,
	or 2 pounds plum tomatoes peeled, seeded and chopped
1	6 ounce (170 g) can tomato paste
1	4 ounce (120 g) can diced green chilies
1	green pepper, chopped
¼	cup chili powder
4	teaspoons ground cumin
1	tablespoon jalapeno chilies, seeded and diced
1	cup (240 ml) water
1	fresh cut pineapple cut into 1-inch cubes
1½	cups, canned white beans (optional), or fresh cooked

Preheat 6-quart (6 L) over medium-high heat for 3-4 minutes. Sprinkle a few drops of water in the pan. If the water droplets dance, the pan is ready. If the water evaporates, the pan is not hot enough. Place the pork in the hot, dry pan, which will be about 400°F (200°C). Cover the pan, and open the vent and dry sauté until browned on all sides, about 10 minutes, stir occasionally. Remove to paper towel to drain.

To the 6-quart, add onions and garlic, sauté until tender, stir occasionally, about 3-4 minutes. Add remaining ingredients, reduce the heat to low, cover with the vent closed, and simmer 2½ hours.

To serve, spoon into individual serving bowls, serve with cornbread (see recipe page 165)

NUTRITIONAL BREAKDOWN PER SERVING: Calories 247; Fat Grams 11; Carbohydrate Grams 24; Protein Grams 14; Cholesterol mg 35; Sodium mg 230 (138 mg with fresh plum tomatoes).

THE POINT SYSTEM: Calorie Points 3 ½; Protein Points 2; Fat Grams 11; Sodium Points 10 (7 points with fresh plum tomatoes); Fiber Points 3; Carbohydrate Points 1½; Cholesterol Points 3.

Blarney Stone Stew

Serves: 12

Preparation Time: 1½ hours

Equipment: French chef knife, cutting board, Kitchen Machine food cutter, 4-quart stockpot

2	pounds (920 g) beef stew meat, trim fat, and cut into 1-inch (2.5 cm) cubes
2	cups (480 ml) dry red wine
2	cloves garlic, minced
½	teaspoon fresh rosemary, finely minced (or dried, crushed)
½	teaspoon fresh thyme, finely minced (or dried, crushed)
2	teaspoons orange zest, grated blade #1
¼	teaspoon pepper
½	cup (120 ml) water
6	carrots, waffle cut blade #5
6	pearl onions, peeled and halved
6	red or new potatoes, quartered
1	cup fresh mushrooms, sliced blade #4 (to slice, lay sideways in hopper)
¼	head red cabbage, shredded blade #5
1	green pepper, chopped
1	15 ounce (425 g) can stewed tomatoes
	or 1¼ pounds plum tomatoes, peeled, seeded and chopped
2	tablespoons cornstarch
2	tablespoons cold water

Preheat skillet over medium-high heat for 3-4 minutes. Place the stew beef in the hot, dry skillet, which will be about 400°F (200°C). Cover the pan, open the vent, and brown until stew beef releases easily from the pan, 4 to 5 minutes. Turn the stew beef and repeat the process until beef is lightly browned on all sides. Drain excess grease from the pan.

To deglaze the skillet, add wine, garlic, rosemary, thyme, orange zest, pepper, ½ cup water. Bring to a simmer, reduce the heat to low, cover with the vent open and simmer one hour.

Add carrots, onions, potatoes, mushrooms, and tomatoes, cover and simmer 30-40 minutes until meat and vegetables are tender. Mix cornstarch and water, add and stir until stew thickens.

To serve, ladle stew into individual serving bowl, top with snipped parsley, and serve with Irish Soda bread (see recipe page 188).

NUTRITIONAL BREAKDOWN PER SERVING: Calories 252; Fat Grams 4; Carbohydrate Grams 26; Protein Grams 22; Cholesterol mg 47; Sodium mg 176.

THE POINT SYSTEM: Calorie Points 3 ½; Protein Points 3; Fat Grams 4; Sodium Points 8; Fiber Points 2; Carbohydrate Points 1½; Cholesterol Points 5.

Marinated Flank Steak

Serves: 8
Preparation Time: 40 minutes
Equipment: French chef knife, cutting board, baking dish, large skillet

2	pounds (1 kg) flank steak
2	cloves garlic, minced
¼	cup onion, minced
¼	cup (60 ml) olive oil
1	fresh lemon, juice of
½	cup (120 ml) red wine
3	tablespoons balsamic vinegar
1	tablespoon dried oregano
1	tablespoon fresh parsley, chopped fine (or dried)

Using a knife, lightly score flank steak, against the grain, on both sides.

To prepare the marinade, in a large baking dish combine garlic, onion, olive oil, lemon juice, red wine, balsamic vinegar, oregano, and parsley. Place the steak in the dish, turning to coat, cover and refrigerate until ready to cook, 20 minutes to an hour. To marinate overnight, place steak in large Zip Lock baggy with marinade and refrigerate. Turn bag occasionally to coat.

Preheat skillet over medium-high heat for 3-4 minutes. Sprinkle a few drops of water in the pan. If the water droplets dance, the pan is ready. If the water evaporates, the pan is not hot enough. Place the steak in the hot, dry skillet, which will be about 400°F (200°C). Cover the pan, and open the vent and brown until steak releases easily from the pan, 4 to 5 minutes. Turn the steak, cover the pan and brown on other side until beef release easily from the skillet, 4 to 5 minutes. (Test for desired doneness as described on page 19). Set aside and allow to rest, 4 to 5 minutes.

For sauce, deglaze skillet with marinade, simmer over medium heat until heated through.

To serve, slice steak diagonally across the grain in ¼-inch (1 cm) strips. Place on serving platter, and drizzle marinade sauce over the steak and serve with asparagus and sweet potatoes cooked the waterless way.

NUTRITIONAL BREAKDOWN PER SERVING: Calories 440; Fat Grams 25; Carbohydrate Grams 5; Protein Grams 44; Cholesterol mg 75; Sodium mg 110.

THE POINT SYSTEM: Calorie Points 6; Protein Points 5½; Fat Grams 25; Sodium Points 5; Fiber Points 0; Carbohydrate Points 0; Cholesterol Points 7½.

Meatloaf

On top of the stove
Serves: 8
Preparation Time: 1 hour
Equipment: French chef knife, cutting board, Kitchen Machine food cutter, large stainless
mixing bowl, large skillet

1½	pounds (700 g) lean ground beef, veal, pork, chicken, turkey, or a combination
½	medium onion, halved, peeled and chopped, blade #3
½	green pepper, chopped
1	stalk celery, chopped or grated, blade #2
1	cup Italian breadcrumbs or oatmeal
½	teaspoon dried or fresh copped oregano
1	teaspoon dried of fresh chopped basil
1	egg or 2 egg whites

In a large mixing bowl, combine all the ingredients, and mix well. Press meatloaf mix into large skillet. Cover, close the vent, and cook over medium-low heat 35-45 minutes.

Variation: top meatloaf mix with sharp cheese, grated #3 blade, and ketchup or tomato sauce. Cook as directed above.

NOTE: If you are limiting the consumption of meat in your diet, our Meatloaf recipe is a wonderful opportunity to substitute TVP (Textured Vegetable protein). Check with you local food store for availability.

To serve, slice meatloaf into 8 equal portions and plate. Serve with waterless cooked vegetables.

Nutritional breakdown does not include cheese, ketchup or tomato sauce

NUTRITIONAL BREAKDOWN PER SERVING: Calories 229; Fat Grams 12; Carbohydrate Grams 12; Protein Grams 17; Cholesterol mg 53; Sodium mg 441

THE POINT SYSTEM: Calorie Points 3; Protein Points 2; Fat Grams 12; Sodium Points 19; Fiber Points 0; Carbohydrate Points 1; Cholesterol Points 5.

Basic Lasagna

On top of the Stove
Serves: 16
Preparation Time: 1 hour
Equipment: French chef knife, Cutting Board, Kitchen Machine food cutter,
12-inch electric skillet or large skillet

4	cups (1 L) Meat Sauce (see page 97)
1	8 ounce (230 g) box lasagna noodle, uncooked
16	ounce (460 g) carton low-fat ricotta cheese
2	cups skim milk mozzarella cheese, shredded blade #3
½	cup Parmesan cheese, grated blade #1

To begin; cover the bottom of the skillet with meat sauce, and place one layer of uncooked lasagna noodles on top of meat sauce. Continue layering in the following order: 1 cup meat sauce, the ricotta cheese, 1 cup mozzarella cheese, 1 cup meat sauce, another layer of lasagna noodles, 1 cup sauce, 1 cup mozzarella, and finally Parmesan cheese on top. Cover:

FOR ELECTRIC SKILLET:
Adjust the electric probe to 225°F (110°C) and bake for 35-45 minutes. Unplug, uncover, and let stand for 10 minutes before serving.

FOR LARGE SKILLET or 13-inch CHEF PAN:
Cover and close the vent, turn heat to medium for 5 minutes, then reduce to low-heat and cook for 35-40 minutes. Remove from heat, uncover and let stand 10 minutes before serving.

To serve, using a serrated knife or spatula, cut into 16 equal portions. Remove lasagna with a flexible spatula and place on individual serving plate. Serve with Garlic Bread, recipe on page 179.

NUTRITIONAL BREAKDOWN PER SERVING: Calories 310; Fat Grams 16; Carbohydrate Grams 17; Protein Grams 25; Cholesterol mg 66; Sodium mg 534.

THE POINT SYSTEM: Calorie Points 4; Protein Points 3; Fat Grams 16; Sodium Points 23; Fiber Points 0; Carbohydrate Points 1; Cholesterol Points 7

Meat Sauce

Serves: 8

Preparation Time: 35 minutes

Equipment: French chef knife, cutting board, Kitchen Machine food cutter, 6-quart 6tockpot

1	tablespoon olive oil
1	onion, halved, peeled and chopped blade #3
2	cloves garlic, minced
2	pounds (1 kg) lean ground beef
1	28 ounce (800 g) can plum tomatoes, diced
	or 2 pounds fresh plum tomatoes, peeled, seeded and chopped
1	12 ounce (350 g) can tomato sauce
3	tablespoons Italian seasoning
2	tablespoons raw sugar (optional)

Preheat 6-quart stockpot over medium-high heat for 3-4 minutes. Add olive oil, bring to temperature, and add onion, sauté 2 to 3 minutes, stirring. Add garlic, sauté 2 to 3 to minutes, or until onion is translucent. Add ground beef, stir to combine with onion and garlic, and stir occasionally until beef is cooked through. Add all other ingredients, reduce to low-heat, cover, close the vent, and simmer 15-20 minutes.

To serve, ladle sauce over your favorite pasta or use in Basic Lasagna recipe on page 96.

Nutritional breakdown includes 2 tablespoons sugar. Sodium in nutritional breakdown is reduced by about 40% if using fresh plum tomatoes.

NUTRITIONAL BREAKDOWN PER SERVING: Calories 261; Fat Grams 15; Carbohydrate Grams 10; Protein Grams 21; Cholesterol mg 70; Sodium mg 154.

THE POINT SYSTEM: Calorie Points 3½; Protein Points 2½; Fat Grams 15; Sodium Points 6½; Fiber Points 1; Carbohydrate Points ½; Cholesterol Points 7.

BBQ Baby Back Ribs

Serves: 10

Preparation Time: 3 hours

Equipment: French chef knife, cutting board, Kitchen Machine food cutter, 6-quart pasta/
steamer basket, 6.5-quart tall stockpot, 3-quart saucepan, 13-inch chef pan

6	pounds (3 kg) baby back pork loin ribs

BRAISING MIXTURE:

5	quarts (5 L) water
1	onion, cut into 1-inch (2.5 cm) chunks
4	celery ribs cut into 1-inch (2.5 cm) chunks
2	cups (480 ml) Burgundy cooking wine

BARBEQUE SAUCE

½	cup green pepper, chopped
1	onion, halved, peeled and chopped blade #3
¼	cup (60 ml) water
1½	cups brown sugar (variation, 1 cup raw sugar)
1	cup molasses
1	cup (60 ml) mustard
2	tablespoons Crystal or Tabasco hot sauce
¼	teaspoon liquid smoke
2	teaspoons Worcestershire sauce
2	cups (480 ml) prepared barbecue sauce
1¼	cups (420 ml) ketchup

Place ribs in 6-quart basket inserted into 6.5-quart stockpot; add water, onion, celery and burgundy wine. Bring to a boil over medium-high heat. Skim froth, reduce to medium-low heat, cover, open vent, and simmer 1½ hours or until meat is tender and pulls easily from the bones.

To prepare BBQ sauce, in the 3-quart dry sauté pepper and onion over medium heat, 3 to 4 minutes, stirring until onion is translucent. Add all other ingredients, stir to combine, reduce the heat to low, cover, close vent, and simmer 45 minutes, stir occasionally.

When ribs are tender, drain and remove from basket, set aside to dry. Preheat oven to 350°F (180°C). Brush ribs with BBQ sauce, and place in 13-inch Chef Pan. Bake in oven 15-20 minutes or until ribs are glazed and candied, brush with BBQ sauce as needed.

To serve, place ribs on large serving platter, whole or sliced, with BBQ sauce on side for dipping.

NUTRITIONAL BREAKDOWN PER SERVING: Calories 551; Fat Grams 27; Carbohydrate Grams 46; Protein Grams 26; Cholesterol mg 62; Sodium mg 608.

THE POINT SYSTEM: Calorie Points 7½; Protein Points 3; Fat Grams 27; Sodium Points 26½; Fiber Points 0; Carbohydrate Points 3; Cholesterol Points 6.

Beef Fajitas

Serves: 12

Preparation Time: 1 hour, 15 minutes

Equipment: French chef knife, cutting board, large stainless mixing bowl, 13-inch chef pan

MARINADE

4	cloves garlic, minced and mashed into a paste, sprinkled with salt
¼	cup (60 ml) fresh squeezed lime juice
1½	teaspoons, ground cumin
2	tablespoons olive oil

FAJITAS

2	pounds (1 kg) flank steak
2	tablespoons vegetable oil, olive oil or sesame seed oil
3	assorted colored bell pepper, sliced thin
1	large red onion, sliced thin
2	garlic cloves, minced
12	7-inch flour tortillas, warmed (see flour tortillas, next recipe)

In the large mixing bowl, prepare marinade by whisking together the garlic paste, lime juice, cumin, and oil. Add the flank steak to the marinade, turning to coat it well, cover and chill in the refrigerator for at least 1 hour, or overnight in Zip Lock baggy, turn occasionally.

To grill the steak, preheat the 13-inch chef pan over medium-high heat. Add steak whole to pan and sear, about 4-5 minutes, turn when it releases easily from the pan and sear the other side. Test for desired doneness (see page 19), and transfer steak to cutting board to rest for about 10 minutes.

Reheat the 13-inch skillet over medium-high heat until it is hot but not smoking; add the bell peppers, onion and garlic. Sauté the mixture, stirring occasionally until the bell peppers are softened, 5-7 minutes

To serve, slice the steak thin across the grain on a diagonal bias and arrange slices on serving platter, topped with bell pepper mixture. Serve with tortillas (see recipe page 100), guacamole (see recipe page 101), and salsa (see recipe page 102).

NUTRITIONAL BREAKDOWN PER SERVING: Calories 542; Fat Grams 21; Carbohydrate Grams 46; Protein Grams 41; Cholesterol mg 75; Sodium mg 394.

THE POINT SYSTEM: Calorie Points 7; Protein Points 5; Fat Grams 21; Sodium Points 17; Fiber Points 1; Carbohydrate Points 3; Cholesterol Points 7.

Flour Tortillas

Yields: 12-7 (18 cm) inch tortillas
Preparation Time: 45-50 minutes
Equipment: French chef knife, cutting board, large stainless mixing bowl,
small stainless mixing bowl, 10-inch gourmet chef pan

TORTILLAS

2	cups all-purpose-flour
¼	cup cold vegetable shortening cut into piece
1	teaspoon salt
⅔	cups warm water

In the large Mixing Bowl blend flour and shortening until the mixture resembles a meal.

In the small Mixing Bowl stir together salt and ⅔ cups warm water, add warm water to flour mixture and toss mixture until water is incorporated. Form dough into a ball and knead it on a lightly floured surface for 2-3 minutes, or until smooth. Divide dough into 12 equal pieces; roll each piece into a ball, and let dough stand, covered with plastic wrap, for at least 20 minutes.

On a lightly floured surface roll one ball of dough at a time into a 7 to 8 inch round.

Preheat 10-inch chef pan over medium-high heat for about 2-3 minutes. Place the tortilla in the pan, turning it ounce, for 1-2 minutes or until it is puffy and golden on both sides. Remove and wrap tortilla in a kitchen towel. Repeat the process of rolling and cooking with the remaining tortillas. Continue to wrap each one, stacking and enclosing them in a towel as they are done. Tortillas may be made in advance and kept chilled in a Zip Lock bag.

To Warm Tortillas: If tortillas are very dry, pat each tortilla between dampened hands before stacking. Stack in skillet, cover, and place over warm burner 10 minutes.

To Assemble Fajitas: Spread guacamole on tortilla, top with sliced steak, bell pepper mixture and salsa. Roll tortilla to enclose filling.

NUTRITIONAL BREAKDOWN PER SERVING: Calories 114; Fat Grams 4; Carbohydrate Grams 16; Protein Grams 2; Cholesterol mg 0; Sodium mg 178.

THE POINT SYSTEM: Calorie Points 1½; Protein Points 0; Fat Grams 4; Sodium Points 8; Fiber Points 0; Carbohydrate Points 1; Cholesterol Points 0.

Guacamole

Serves: 8
Preparation Time: 15 minutes
Equipment: French chef knife, cutting board, medium stainless mixing bowl

2	ripe avocados
1	small onion, minced fine
1	clove garlic, minced and using the side of the knife, mashed into a paste
1	fresh lime, juice thereof
½	teaspoon ground cumin
1	plum tomato, peeled, seeded and diced
3	tablespoons fresh coriander, chopped or cilantro

Halve and pit the avocados and scoop the flesh into a bowl. Mash avocados with a fork and stir in onion, garlic paste, lime juice, cumin, tomato, and coriander.

NOTE: Guacamole can be prepared in advance and kept chilled and covered.

NUTRITIONAL BREAKDOWN PER SERVING: Calories 62; Fat Grams 5; Carbohydrate Grams 5; Protein Grams 1; Cholesterol mg 0; Sodium mg 8.

THE POINT SYSTEM: Calorie Points 1; Protein Points 0; Fat Grams 5; Sodium Points 0; Fiber Points ½; Carbohydrate Points ½; Cholesterol Points 0.

Tomato Salsa

Serves: 8
Preparation Time: 15 minutes
Equipment: French chef knife, cutting board, medium stainless mixing bowl

1	pound (460 g) plum tomatoes, peeled, seeded and chopped (instructions below)
1	small onion, minced fine
1	tablespoon lime juice, fresh squeezed
2	tablespoons fresh coriander, chopped (optional)
1	jalapeno chili, seeded and minced

In a mixing bowl, toss together tomatoes, onion, lime juice, coriander, and jalapeno. Allow salsa stand for about 30 minutes.

NOTE: Salsa may be made in advance, keep covered and chilled. However, salsa is best served at room temperature.

NUTRITIONAL BREAKDOWN PER SERVING: Calories 22; Fat Grams 0; Carbohydrate Grams 5; Protein Grams 1; Cholesterol mg 0; Sodium mg 16.

THE POINT SYSTEM: Calorie Points ½; Protein Points 0; Fat Grams 0; Sodium Points 1; Fiber Points ½; Carbohydrate Points ½; Cholesterol Points 0.

How to Peel & Seed Tomatoes

Equipment: large mixing bowl, 4-quart stockpot, paring knife, slotted serving spoon, large mixing bowl

In the mixing bowl, prepare an ice bath of ice and water. Add ice as needed to stay cold.

Fill the 4-quart halfway water and bring to a boil over medium-high heat. With a paring knife score an X across the top stem of the tomatoes. Using a slotted with long handle, place tomatoes in boiling water, 1 to 2 minutes, or until the skin at the X begins to peel back slightly. Using the slotted spoon, quickly remove tomato to ice bath.

Using the Paring knife, beginning at the X, peel the skin from the tomato. With a French chef knife slice the tomato in half and scoop out the seeds with a tablespoon.

Plum tomatoes peeled and seeded can be used in a variety of tomato based recipes.

Stuffed Cabbage Rolls

Serves: 6
Preparation Time: 1 hour, 15 minutes
Equipment: French chef knife, cutting board, Kitchen Machine food cutter, 6.5-quart stockpot,
6-quart steamer/pasta Basket, large stainless mixing bowl, large skillet, small stainless mixing bowl

FILLING

6	large green cabbage leaves
½	pound (230 g) ground turkey
½	pound (230 g) lean ground pork or veal
1	cup cooked rice
½	medium onion, halved, peeled and chopped blade #3
½	teaspoon fresh basil, minced (or dried)
½	teaspoon fresh parsley, minced (or dried)
½	teaspoon fresh oregano, minced (or dried)
½	small garlic clove, minced and mashed into a paste with side of chef's knife

Pinch black ground pepper and kosher or sea salt to taste (optional)

SAUCE

1	8 ounce (230 g) can tomato sauce
	or ¾ pound plum tomatoes peeled, seeded and chopped
½	teaspoon fresh basil, minced (or dried)
½	teaspoon fresh parsley, minced (or dried)
½	teaspoon fresh oregano, minced (or dried)

In the 6.5-quart stockpot with steamer/pasta basket inserted, add 2-3 cups of water and bring to a boil. Place cabbage leaves in basket, cover, open the vent, and steam cabbage until leaves wilt, approximately 7-10 minutes. Set aside to cool.

In the large Mixing Bowl, combine turkey, pork (or veal) rice, and spices, mix well. Place ½ cup of mixture in the center of each cabbage leaf, fold ends of leaf over mixture and roll up. Place cabbage rolls in cold large skillet folded seam side down.

In the small mixing bowl, combine sauce ingredients and pour evenly over cabbage rolls. Cover, close the vent, and cook over medium-low heat, 30-35 minutes.

NUTRITIONAL BREAKDOWN PER SERVING: Calories 188; Fat Grams 8; Carbohydrate Grams 12; Protein Grams 17; Cholesterol mg 55; Sodium mg 124.

THE POINT SYSTEM: Calorie Points 2½; Protein Points 2; Fat Grams 8; Sodium Points 5; Fiber Points 0; Carbohydrate Points 1; Cholesterol Points 5.

Stuffed Peppers

Serves: 4

Preparation Time: 1 hour

Equipment: French chef knife, cutting board, Kitchen Machine food cutter,
large skillet, 4-quart stockpot

4	medium green bell peppers
½	medium onion, peeled and chopped blade #3
1	celery rib, chopped
1	clove garlic, minced
1	tablespoon olive oil
½	pound (230 g) lean ground round
1	cup cooked rice
1	8 ounce (230 g) can tomato sauce
	or ¾ pound plum tomatoes peeled, seeded and chopped
1	2 ½ ounce (75 g) jar sliced mushrooms
½	teaspoon oregano
1	teaspoon fresh basil, chopped (or dried)

With a knife, slice off tops of green peppers and remove seeds. Remove the stem and chop green pepper tops.

In the large skillet over medium heat, dry sauté chopped pepper tops, onions, celery and garlic until tender (olive oil for sautéing optional). Add ground beef, sauté until cooked through. Add all other ingredients and stir until well blended. Remove from heat to cool.

Spoon beef and rice mixture into bell peppers, stand peppers upright in 4-quart stockpot (4 L). Add 3 tablespoons of water to pan, cover with the vent closed, and cook waterless over medium-low heat to form the vapor seal. When the lid spins freely on a cushion of water the vapor seal is formed. Cook through until tender, 20-25 minutes.

NUTRITIONAL BREAKDOWN PER SERVING: Calories 258; Fat Grams 11; Carbohydrate Grams 26; Protein Grams 14; Cholesterol mg 35; Sodium mg 471.

THE POINT SYSTEM: Calorie Points 3½; Protein Points 2; Fat Grams 11; Sodium Points 20½; Fiber Points 2; Carbohydrate Points 2; Cholesterol Points 3.

Sweet & Sour Pork

Serves: 6
Preparation Time: 1 hour, 30 minutes
Equipment: French chef knife, cutting board, 11-inch mini-WOK

1	cup flour
4	tablespoons cornstarch
1½	teaspoons baking powder
1	pinch salt
1	tablespoon oil
	Water
8	ounces (230 g) pork tenderloin cut into ½-inch (1.5 cm) cubes
½	cup oil for frying
1	onion, sliced
1	green bell pepper, cored, seeded and sliced
1	small can pineapple chunks, juice reserved

SWEET AND SOUR SAUCE

2	tablespoons cornstarch
½	cup light brown sugar
1	pinch salt
½	cup (120 ml) apple cider vinegar or rice vinegar
1	clove garlic, crushed
6	tablespoons tomato ketchup
6	tablespoons reserved pineapple juice

To prepare batter, sift flour, cornstarch, baking powder and salt into mixing bowl. Make a well in the center; add oil and enough water to make a thick, smooth batter. Stir well, gradually incorporating flour from the outside, and beat until smooth.

Heat oil in wok over medium-high heat, dip pork into the batter and drop into hot oil. Fry 4-5 pieces of pork at a time until golden brown, remove with slotted spoon to paper towels. Continue until all pork is fried. Pour off oil from the wok; add onion, pepper and pineapple. Stir-fry over medium-high heat for 1-2 minutes. Remove vegetable, pineapple mixture from wok and set aside.

In a mixing bowl, combine sauce ingredients, mix well, pour into wok, and bring to a boil slowly, over medium heat, stirring continuously until mixture thickens. Allow to simmer for 1-2 minutes until clear. Add vegetables, pineapple, and pork cubes to the sauce and stir to coat completely, sauté for 1-2 minutes and serve immediately.

NUTRITIONAL BREAKDOWN PER SERVING: Calories 324; Fat Grams 6; Carbohydrate Grams 57; Protein Grams 12; Cholesterol mg 22; Sodium mg 325.

THE POINT SYSTEM: Calorie Points 4½; Protein Points 1½; Fat Grams 6; Sodium Points 14; Fiber Points 1; Carbohydrate Points 4; Cholesterol Points 2.
Pork and Shrimp Pot Stickers

Pork & Shrimp Pot Stickers

Yields: 48 Pot Stickers, Serves: 12
Time: 1 hour, 15 minutes
Equipment: French chef knife, Cutting Board, Kitchen Machine food cutter, large stainless
Mixing Bowl, medium stainless Mixing Bowl, Large Skillet

3	cups flour
¼	teaspoon salt
1	cup (240 ml) warm water
½	pound (230 g) shrimp, peeled and shelled, chopped fine
½	pound (230 g) ground pork
1	cup green cabbage, chopped #2 blade
3	green onion, minced
¼	cup mushrooms, minced
2	tablespoons soy sauce
1	clove garlic, minced
1 ⅓	cups (320 ml) low sodium chicken broth, divided (or homemade stock)

In large Mixing Bowl combine flour, salt and warm water and mix well. On an un-floured board, knead dough until very smooth and satiny. Cover and let rest for 30 minutes.

In medium Mixing Bowl, combine the shrimp, pork, cabbage, onions, mushrooms, soy sauce and garlic. Mix well.

Divide dough into two portions, keeping half covered to keep from drying out. Roll the dough to about one-eighth (50 mm) inch thickness. Cut our 3-inch (7.5 cm) circles; place the filling in the center of each circle of dough. Fold in half, pinching the edges closed, making a few tucks along the edge. Cover finished pot sticker and complete other half.

Spray large skillet with cooking spray or lightly oil. Preheat the pan over medium heat; place Pot Stickers in pan, cooking 12 at a time. Cook until bottoms are golden brown.

Pour ⅓ cup chicken stock over pot stickers, reduce heat to low, cover with the vent open, and steam for about 15 minutes. Remove cover and transfer pot stickers to plate. Rinse skillet, wipe dry, and repeat process beginning with cooking spray or oiling the skillet.

Serve with Soy Dipping Sauce, see recipe page 159.

NUTRITIONAL BREAKDOWN PER SERVING: Calories 190; Fat Grams 4; Carbohydrate Grams 24; Protein Grams 12; Cholesterol mg 44; Sodium mg 474.

THE POINT SYSTEM: Calorie Points 1; Protein Points 1; Fat Grams 4; Sodium Points 20; Fiber Points 0; Carbohydrate Points 2; Cholesterol Points 4.

Pork and Pumpkin Stew

Serves: 6

Time: 1 hour

Equipment: French chef knife, cutting board, Kitchen Machine food cutter, 6-quart stockpot

1 ½	pound (700 g) pork tenderloin, trimmed and cut 1 ½-inch (4 cm) cubes
2	teaspoons olive oil
2	teaspoons whole cumin seeds
1	large onion, halved, peeled and chopped #3 blade
3	cloves garlic, minced
1	14 ounce (400 g) can crushed tomatoes, or 1½ pounds plum tomatoes, peeled, seeded and chopped
1	cup (240 ml) chicken stock
½	cup (120 ml) dry white wine
½	teaspoon fresh oregano, chopped (or dried)
¼	teaspoon red pepper flakes
1	pound (460 g) fresh pumpkin*, peeled, cut into 1-inch (2.5 cm) chunks (3 cups)
1	tablespoon cornstarch
1	tablespoon water
3	tablespoons fresh parsley or cilantro, chopped
2	tablespoons pumpkin seeds (pepitas) lightly toasted (optional)

Preheat 6-quart Stockpot (6 L) over medium-high heat. Add pork cubes, brown on all sides, remove from pan and set aside. Reduce heat to low, add oil and cumin, sauté 30 seconds, add onion and garlic, sauté 2 minutes. Add tomatoes, chicken stock, wine, oregano, red pepper flakes and reserved pork. Cover, open vent, and simmer over low heat 30 minutes.

Dissolve cornstarch in water, add to stew to thicken, stirring gently. Add cilantro or parsley, and salt and pepper to taste.

To serve, ladle stew into individual serving bowls, and top with toasted pumpkin seeds.

*Butternut squash can be used in place of pumpkin.

NUTRITIONAL BREAKDOWN PER SERVING: Calories 314; Fat Grams 13; Carbohydrate Grams 18; Protein Grams 30; Cholesterol mg 65; Sodium mg 222.

THE POINT SYSTEM: Calorie Points 4; Protein Points 4; Fat Grams 13; Sodium Points 10; Fiber Points 1; Carbohydrate Points 1; Cholesterol Points 6.

Poultry. . .

Lemon Sesame Chicken

Serves: 4
Time: 20 minutes
Equipment: French chef knife, cutting board, large skillet or electric skillet

4	skinless chicken breasts
I	fresh lemon, juice thereof
I	tablespoon sesame seeds
I	teaspoon oregano

Preheat skillet over medium-high heat for 3-4 minutes, electric skillet (350°F/180°C). Sprinkle a few drops of water in the pan. If the water droplets dance, the pan is ready. If the water evaporates, the pan is not hot enough. Place the chicken in the hot, dry pan. Cover the pan, open the vent, and brown chicken until it releases easily from the skillet, 5 to 7 minutes. Turn the chicken, cover the pan and brown, 4 to 5 minutes. Test for doneness.

To serve, sprinkle with fresh lemon juice and top with sesame seeds and oregano.

NUTRITIONAL BREAKDOWN PER SERVING: Calories 304; Fat Grams 7; Carbohydrate Grams 4; Protein Grams 54; Cholesterol mg 146; Sodium mg 127.

THE POINT SYSTEM: Calorie Points 4; Protein Points 7; Fat Grams 7; Sodium Points 6; Fiber Points 0; Carbohydrate Points ½ ; Cholesterol Points 15.

Chicken and Roasted Garlic

Serves: 6

Time: 50 minutes

Equipment: French chef knife, cutting board, 13-inch chef pan

4	pounds (2 kg) bone-in chicken pieces, skinned
40	cloves garlic, unpeeled (about 4 bulbs)
1½	cups (420 ml) dry white wine
¼	teaspoon (4 sprigs) fresh thyme
¼	teaspoon (1 sprig) rosemary
2	tablespoons Cognac
1	tablespoon fresh parsley, chopped
12	slices coarse bread, toasted

Preheat the 13-inch chef pan over medium or medium-high heat, about 3 minutes. Test the surface with a few water droplets. If the droplets bead up and dance across the surface, the pan is hot enough to brown the chicken and seal in juices. Place the chicken in the pan; it will stick at first while browning. Cover the pan and open the vent. When the chicken loosens, about 5-7 minutes, turn it to brown on the other side. About 4-5 minutes. Test for doneness and remove the chicken from the pan.

Add the unpeeled garlic to the Chef's pan and continue stirring for 3-5 minutes until garlic begins to brown. Spread the garlic around the pan evenly and return the chicken pieces to the pan. Add the wine, thyme, and rosemary. Cover with the vent open, reduce to low-heat, and simmer for 20-25 minutes.

Drizzle Cognac over the chicken, cover and continue to simmer for about 5 minutes with the cover off.

To serve, remove the chicken pieces to a serving platter, surround with roasted garlic cloves, top with chopped parsley, and serve with toasted bread.

NOTE: When the garlic is squeezed out of its natural wrapper it spreads like butter on the bread.

NUTRITIONAL BREAKDOWN PER SERVING: Calories 250; Fat Grams 6; Carbohydrate Grams 18; Protein Grams 22; Cholesterol mg 58; Sodium mg 251.

THE POINT SYSTEM: Calorie Points 3; Protein Points 3; Fat Grams 6; Sodium Points 11; Fiber Points 2; Carbohydrate Points 1; Cholesterol Points 6.

Lemon Baked Chicken

Serves: 4

Time: 40 minutes

Equipment: French chef knife, cutting board, large skillet, I-quart stainless mixing bowl

4	chicken breast halves, skinless
3	tablespoon fresh squeezed lemon juice
2	tablespoons water
¼	teaspoon onion powder
¼	teaspoon marjoram leaves
¼	teaspoon sea salt or kosher salt
¼	teaspoon paprika
I	tablespoon fresh parsley, chopped

Preheat the large skillet over medium or medium-high heat, about 3 minutes. Test the surface with a few water droplets. If the droplets bead up and dance across the surface, the pan is hot enough to brown the chicken and seal in juices. Place the chicken in the pan; it will stick at first while browning. Cover the pan and open the vent. When the chicken loosens, about 5-7 minutes, turn it to brown on the other side. About 4-5 minutes. Test for doneness.

In the small mixing bowl, combine all other ingredients, except parsley, and pour over browned chicken. Cover with the vent closed, reduce to low-heat, and simmer 15 minutes.

To serve, remove chicken to individual serving plates, garnish with parsley, and serve with lemon and orange slices. Serve with snow peas with toasted sesame seeds.

NUTRITIONAL BREAKDOWN PER SERVING: Calories 298; Fat Grams 6; Carbohydrate Grams 4; Protein Grams 54; Cholesterol mg 146; Sodium mg 261.

THE POINT SYSTEM: Calorie Points 4; Protein Points 7; Fat Grams 6; Sodium Points 11; Fiber Points 0; Carbohydrate Points 0; Cholesterol Points 15.

Chicken Cacciatore

Serves: 6

Time: 40 minutes

Equipment: French chef knife, cutting board, Kitchen Machine food cutter,
large skillet, 2-quart saucepan

3	whole chicken breasts halved and skinned (or 12 chicken thighs, skin removed)
1	cup uncooked long-grain rice (or brown rice)
2	cups (480 ml) low sodium chicken broth (or homemade chicken stock)
1	cup celery, finely chopped
1	large onion, halved, peeled and chopped blade #3
2	cloves garlic, minced
½	green pepper, chopped
½	sweet red pepper, chopped
7	fresh mushrooms, sliced blade #4 (to slice, place mushrooms sideways in hopper)
1	16 ounce (460 g) can whole tomatoes, halved
	or 1½ pounds fresh plum tomatoes, peeled, seeded and chopped
1	15 ounce (425 g) can tomato sauce or homemade tomato sauce

Preheat the large skillet over medium or medium-high heat, about 3 minutes. Test the surface with a few water droplets. If the droplets bead up and dance across the surface, the pan is hot enough to brown the chicken and seal in juices. Place the chicken in the pan; it will stick at first while browning. Cover the pan and open the vent. When the chicken loosens, about 5-7 minutes, turn it to brown on the other side, about 4-5 minutes. Remove chicken from pan and set aside.

In the 2-quart, bring the chicken stock to a boil over medium-high heat, add rice, stir, cover, close the vent, and reduce to low-heat. Rice should cook through in 30-35 minutes.

To the large skillet, add celery, onion, garlic, green and red peppers, sauté until tender, about 5 minutes. Add the mushrooms and sweat down, about 5 minutes, stirring occasionally. Add the tomatoes, and tomato sauce, and stir into mixture. Place the browned chicken on top, reduce to low-heat, cover with the vent closed, and simmer 15-20 minutes.

To serve, divide rice equally on serving plates, place chicken on rice and top with sauce.

NUTRITIONAL BREAKDOWN PER SERVING: Calories 346; Fat Grams 5; Carbohydrate Grams 45; Protein Grams 35; Cholesterol mg 73; Sodium mg 284 (171 with homemade chicken stock and fresh tomatoes).

THE POINT SYSTEM: Calorie Points 4 ½; Protein Points 4; Fat Grams 5; Sodium Points 12 (7-8 points with homemade chicken stock and fresh tomatoes); Fiber Points 3; Carbohydrate Points 3; Cholesterol Points 7.

Evening Parmesan Chicken

Serves: 6
Time: 45 minutes
Equipment: French chef knife, cutting board, Kitchen Machine food cutter,
large skillet, 2-quart stainless mixing bowl

6	chicken breast halves, skinned with bone in
¼	cup Italian Bread crumbs
½	cup Parmesan cheese, grated blade #1
3	tablespoons fresh parsley, chopped
¼	teaspoon black pepper, freshly grated
½	cup (120 ml) Italian Salad Dressing (see recipe page 71)
2	tablespoons fresh chopped parsley

Preheat the large skillet over medium or medium-high heat, about 3 minutes. Test the surface with a few water droplets. If the droplets bead up and dance across the surface, the pan is hot enough to brown the chicken and seal in juices. Place the chicken in the pan; it will stick at first while browning. Cover the pan and open the vent. When the chicken loosens, about 5-7 minutes, turn it to brown on the other side, about 4-5 minutes. Remove chicken to serving platter.

In 2-quart mixing bowl, combine dry ingredients, and set aside. Brush chicken with salad dressing, then sprinkle bread crumb mixture on chicken. Return chicken to pan, breast meat-side up, cover, open the vent, reduce to low-heat and bake on top of the stove, 20 minutes.

To serve, removed chicken to individual serving plates, top with fresh chopped parsley, and serve with sliced, yellow squash and zucchini cooked the waterless way.

NUTRITIONAL BREAKDOWN PER SERVING: Calories 384; Fat Grams 11; Carbohydrate Grams 11; Protein Grams 57; Cholesterol mg 152; Sodium mg 503.

THE POINT SYSTEM: Calorie Points 5; Protein Points 7; Fat Grams 11; Sodium Points 22; Fiber Points 0; Carbohydrate Points 1; Cholesterol Points 15.

Chicken Thighs Marengo

Serves: 6

Time: 45 minutes

Equipment: French chef knife, cutting board, Kitchen Machine food cutter, large skillet

6	chicken thighs, skinned
1	cup fresh mushrooms, sliced blade #4 (to slice, place sideways in hopper)
4	green onions, chopped
1	clove garlic, minced
½	cup (120 ml) Chablis or other dry white wine
1	teaspoon fresh thyme, chopped or ¼ teaspoon dried
2	medium tomatoes cut into wedges
1	tablespoon fresh parsley, chopped

Preheat the large skillet over medium or medium-high heat, about 3 minutes. Test the surface with a few water droplets. If the droplets bead up and dance across the surface, the pan is hot enough to brown the chicken and seal in juices. Place the chicken in the pan; it will stick at first while browning. Cover the pan and open the vent. When the chicken loosens, about 5-7 minutes, turn it to brown on the other side, about 4-5 minutes. Remove chicken to serving platter.

Add mushrooms to skillet, and sweat down, stirring 2-3 minutes. Remove mushrooms and set aside.

Add onions and garlic to pan and sauté until tender, 4-5 minutes. Deglaze skillet with wine, stir in thyme, return the chicken to then pan, and bring to a simmer. Reduce to low-heat, cover, close the vent, and cook 15-20 minutes.

Add tomatoes, and return the mushrooms to the skillet, cover, close the vent, and cook 2-3 minutes.

To serve, place chicken thighs in six individual serving bowls, spoon tomato and mushroom mixture over chicken, top with chopped parsley and serve.

NUTRITIONAL BREAKDOWN PER SERVING: Calories 136; Fat Grams 6; Carbohydrate Grams 3; Protein Grams 14; Cholesterol mg 49; Sodium mg 52.

THE POINT SYSTEM: Calorie Points 2; Protein Points 2; Fat Grams 6; Sodium Points 2; Fiber Points 0; Carbohydrate Points 0; Cholesterol Points 5.

Roasted Chicken with Rosemary

Serves: 4-6
Time: 1 hour, 20 minutes
Equipment: French chef knife, cutting board, 8-quart stockpot

1	whole chicken
3	sprigs fresh rosemary
¼	cup olive oil

Clean chicken, and place whole sprig of rosemary in cavity and one in fold of each wing, next to the breast. (Tie chicken with string to keep rosemary in place, and wings tucked). Baste chicken with olive oil.

Place chicken on its side in 8-quart Stockpot. Cover, close the vent, and roast over low-heat 30 minutes. Turn the chicken to the other side, cover, and roast an additional 30 minutes. Turn chicken upright, and roast an additional 20 minutes.

If desired, increase to medium-high heat and deglaze the stockpot with 2 cups chicken stock and ¼ cup white wine. Reduce liquid by half to thicken, or add or 1 tablespoon cornstarch mixed with 1 tablespoon water to thicken.

To serve, slice chicken and serve with rice and gravy.

NUTRITIONAL BREAKDOWN PER SERVING: Calories 364; Fat Grams 25; Carbohydrate Grams 2; Protein Grams 31; Cholesterol mg 121; Sodium mg 84.

THE POINT SYSTEM: Calorie Points 5; Protein Points 4; Fat Grams 25; Sodium Points 4; Fiber Points 0; Carbohydrate Points 0; Cholesterol Points 12.

Chicken Tikka

Serves: 6
Time: 15 minutes (marinate 2 hours)
Equipment: French chef knife, cutting board, Kitchen Machine food cutter,
large stainless mixing bowl, large skillet

CHICKEN

3	boneless, skinless, chicken breasts
3	legs and thighs, skinned

MARINADE

I	teaspoon paprika
½	teaspoon cayenne pepper
I	teaspoon raw sugar
I	teaspoon pepper, freshly ground
I	teaspoon cumin, freshly ground
I	teaspoon coriander, freshly ground
3	cloves garlic, minced
I	teaspoon fresh ginger, grated blade #I
3	tablespoons vinegar
2	tablespoons ketchup
2	tablespoons olive oil

With a chef knife, score chicken to the bone every ½-inch (1.5 cm).

In the large mixing bowl, combine the marinade ingredients. Mix well and add chicken to the marinade, cover and refrigerate 2 hours, or overnight in a Zip Lock baggy, turn occasionally.

To cook, preheat the large skillet over medium or medium-high heat, about 3 minutes. Test the surface with a few water droplets. If the droplets bead up and dance across the surface, the pan is hot enough to brown the chicken and seal in juices. Place the chicken in the pan; it will stick at first while browning. Cover the pan and open the vent. When the chicken loosens, about 5-7 minutes, turn it to brown on the other side, about 4-5 minutes. Remove chicken to serving platter.

To serve, add remaining marinade to skillet, and cook about 5 minutes. Pour sauce over chicken and serve with Roasted Pepper Salad, recipe page 62.

NUTRITIONAL BREAKDOWN PER SERVING: Calories 286; Fat Grams 12; Carbohydrate Grams 3; Protein Grams 40; Cholesterol mg 118; Sodium mg 141.

THE POINT SYSTEM: Calorie Points 4; Protein Points 5; Fat Grams 12; Sodium Points 6; Fiber Points 0; Carbohydrate Points 0; Cholesterol Points 12.

Chicken Satay with Peanut Sauce

Serves: 8
Preparation Time: 1 hour, 15 minutes
Equipment: French chef knife, cutting board, 7-inch chef ran, rectangular baking dish, small
stainless mixing bowl, 2 burner double griddle

1	package (16) bamboo skewers
1 ½	teaspoons fennel seed
2	teaspoons ground turmeric
2	pounds (1 kg) boneless, skinless chicken breasts
¼	cup (180 ml) unsweetened coconut milk
1	tablespoon soy sauce

Soak skewers in water 10-15 minutes.

In the 7-inch Chef Pan, dry roast fennel seeds until light brown. Grind fennel seed and turmeric together with a mortar and pestle or a coffee grinder used only for spices.

Using the French chef knife, slice chicken into ½-inch (1.5 cm) strips, the full length of the breast. Ribbon thread chicken onto 16 skewers, and place in rectangular baking dish.

In small mixing bowl combine coconut milk, soy sauce and ground spices. Pour over chicken to coat. Marinate 1 hour in refrigerator, cover, and turn occasionally.

To cook, preheat the double griddle over medium or medium-high heat, about 3 minutes. Test the surface with a few water droplets. If the droplets bead up and dance across the surface, the pan is hot enough to brown the chicken and seal in juices. Place the chicken skewers on the griddle; it will stick at first while browning. When the chicken loosens, about 3-5 minutes, turn it to brown on the other side. Continue searing until all sides are browned and chicken is cooked through. About 3-5 minutes per side.

To serve, serve with Chinese "not fried" rice, recipe page 173, and Peanut Sauce, recipe page 118.

NUTRITIONAL BREAKDOWN PER SERVING: Calories 340; Fat Grams 12; Carbohydrate Grams 2; Protein Grams 54; Cholesterol mg 146; Sodium mg 259.

THE POINT SYSTEM: Calorie Points 5; Protein Points 7; Fat Grams 12; Sodium Points 11; Fiber Points 0; Carbohydrate Points 0; Cholesterol Points 15.

Peanut Sauce

Yields 1 1/2 cups
Serving Size: 1 tablespoon
Preparation Time: 15 minutes
Equipment: French chef knife, cutting board, Kitchen Machine food cutter,
small stainless mixing bowl

½   cup peanut butter
¼   cup (60 ml) warm water
¼   cup (60 ml) rice wine vinegar
1   clove garlic, minced fine and mashed into a paste with side of knife
½   tablespoon ginger, freshly grated blade #1
1   teaspoon raw sugar
1   teaspoon red chili flakes
¼   cup (60 ml) sesame oil

In a mixing bowl, using a whisk, thin the peanut butter by stirring in warm water slowly. Whisk in all other ingredients except for sesame oil. Slowly blend in sesame oil by pouring a very thin stream of oil as you continue to whisk the peanut sauce.

To serve, sauce can be served at room temperature with Chicken Satay or hot.

NUTRITIONAL BREAKDOWN PER SERVING: Calories 36; Fat Grams 3; Carbohydrate Grams 2; Protein Grams 1; Cholesterol mg 0; Sodium mg 31.

THE POINT SYSTEM: Calorie Points ½; Protein Points 2; Fat Grams 3; Sodium Points 1½; Fiber Points 0; Carbohydrate Points 0; Cholesterol Points 0.

Ground Turkey Stuffed Peppers

Serves: 4

Preparation Time: 50 minutes

Equipment: French chef knife, cutting board, Kitchen Machine food cutter,
2-quart saucepan, large skillet

1½	cups (360 ml) chicken broth or homemade chicken stock
¾	cup rice
1	tablespoon olive oil
1	onion, halved, peeled and chopped blade #3
2	cloves garlic, minced
1½	pound pounds (700 g) ground turkey
1	32 ounce (910 g) can tomato sauce
4	tablespoons fresh parsley, chopped
1	teaspoon sea salt or kosher salt
½	teaspoon fresh ground pepper
6	large green bell peppers

In the 2-quart saucepan (2 L) bring chicken stock to a boil, add rice, stir, cover, close vent, and remove from heat.

In 8-inch chef pan, over medium-high heat, sauté onion and garlic in olive oil 3-5 minutes. Add ground turkey, and cook until turkey is no longer pink in color. Drain liquid, if any. Stir in cooked rice, tomato sauce, parsley, salt and pepper, and mix well.

Remove tops and seed green peppers. Spoon turkey and rice mixture into bell peppers and stand peppers upright in large skillet. Spoon remaining sauce on top of pepper, and add 3 tablespoons of water to skillet, cover, close the vent, and cook waterless over medium-low heat to form the vapor seal. When the lid spins freely on a cushion of water the vapor seal is formed. Cook through until tender, approximately 25 minutes.

NUTRITIONAL BREAKDOWN PER SERVING: Calories 320; Fat Grams 13; Carbohydrate Grams 26; Protein Grams 26; Cholesterol mg 90; Sodium mg 165.

THE POINT SYSTEM: Calorie Points 4½; Protein Points 3; Fat Grams 13; Sodium Points 7; Fiber Points 3; Carbohydrate Points 1½; Cholesterol Points 9.

Chicken Enchiladas

Serves: 8
Preparation Time: 1 hour
Equipment: French chef knife, cutting board, Kitchen Machine food cutter,
6-quart steamer/pasta basket, 6½ -quart stockpot, medium stainless mixing bowl,
electric food processor, 13-inch chef pan

2	whole chicken breasts, bone in with skin
1	onion, quartered
1	bay leaf
8	pepper whole corns
3	tablespoons Parmesan cheese, grated #1 blade
½	cup Monterey Jack cheese, shredded #2 blade
1	4.5-ounce (125 g) can green chilies
1	15-ounce (425 g) canned tomatoes, drained
	or 1¼ pounds plum tomatoes, peeled and seeded
¼	cup cilantro
½	cup (120 ml) buttermilk
8	corn tortillas
½	cup cheddar cheese

Place chicken breasts, onion, bay leaf and pepper corns in the 6-quart steamer/pasta basket inserted in 6½ stockpot, and cover with water, open the vent, and simmer over low-heat 30 minutes. Cool in refrigerator.

Shred chicken, discarding bones, skin and basket contents, reserve chicken broth for future use. In the mixing bowl combine chicken with Parmesan and Monterey Jack cheese. Set aside.

In the food processor, combine green chilies, tomatoes, cilantro, and butter milk, and set aside.

To soften tortillas, place between damp paper towels in 13-inch (33 cm) chef pan, cover, close vent, and place over low-heat, 5-7 minutes. Fill each tortilla with one-eighth of the chicken and cheese mixture. Roll tightly.

Place the tortillas seam-side down in the 13-inch chef pan. Add chili-tomato mixture, cover open the vent, and simmer over medium-low heat 20-25 minutes.

To serve, before removing from pan, sprinkle with cheddar cheese. If desired, top Low-fat sour cream and chopped black olives.

NUTRITIONAL BREAKDOWN PER SERVING: Calories 202; Fat Grams 5; Carbohydrate Grams 18; Protein Grams 22; Cholesterol mg 44; Sodium mg 250.

THE POINT SYSTEM: Calorie Points 2½; Protein Points 3; Fat Grams 5; Sodium Points 11; Fiber Points 1; Carbohydrate Points 1; Cholesterol Points 4.

Teriyaki Chicken

Serves: 8
Preparation Time: 45 minutes
Equipment: French chef knife, cutting board, Kitchen Machine food cutter,
medium stainless Mixing bowl, 11-inch mini/WOK

2	boneless, skinless chicken breasts, sliced into ½-inch (1.5 cm) strips
¼	cup brown sugar, or raw sugar
¼	cup (60 ml) rice wine vinegar
2	tablespoons soy sauce
1	tablespoon fresh ginger, grated blade #1
1	clove garlic, minced
1	onion, sliced
1	green pepper, sliced
1	red pepper, sliced
1	cup fresh pineapple, cubed

In the mixing bowl, combine chicken, brown sugar, vinegar, soy sauce, ginger and garlic. Cover and Marinade chicken ½ hour.

Preheat wok over medium-high heat, add chicken strips and stir-fry 3-4 minutes, add onions, peppers, and pineapple, stir fry 2-3 minutes. Add marinade and reduce to low-heat, cover with the vent open, and simmer about 5 minutes, or until chicken is cooked through but tender.

Serve over rice or rice noodles.

NUTRITIONAL BREAKDOWN PER SERVING: Calories 259; Fat Grams 4; Carbohydrate Grams 28; Protein Grams 29; Cholesterol mg 73; Sodium mg 587.

THE POINT SYSTEM: Calorie Points 3½; Protein Points 4; Fat Grams 4; Sodium Points 26; Fiber Points 1; Carbohydrate Points 2; Cholesterol Points 7.

Turkey with Orzo and Broccoli

Serves: 8
Preparation Time: 30 minutes
Equipment: French chef knife, cutting board, 13-inch chef pan

I	skinless turkey breasts, cut into strips
I	onion, sliced thin
3	cloves garlic, chopped
I	16 ounce (460 g) can chopped tomatoes
	or 1½ pounds plum tomatoes, peeled, seeded and chopped
1½	cups uncooked orzo pasta
2	cups (480 ml) water, or chicken broth
I	medium head fresh broccoli florets

Preheat 13-inch (33 cm) chef pan over medium or medium-high heat, about 3 minutes. Test the surface with a few water droplets. If the droplets bead up and dance across the surface, the pan is hot enough to brown the turkey and seal in juices. Place the turkey strips in the pan; it will stick at first while browning. Cover the pan and open the vent. When the turkey loosens, about 3-5 minutes, turn it to brown on the other side. About 4-5 minutes.

Add onion and garlic, sauté 2-3 minutes. Reduce to medium-low heat, add tomatoes and mix well. Push mixture to center of pan. Pour dried orzo around outside rim of pan, pour water over orzo, cover, close vent, and cook 10 minutes; top with broccoli, cover and cook about 5 minutes.

To serve, place hot 13-inch chef pan on trivet and serve directly from pan.

NUTRITIONAL BREAKDOWN PER SERVING: Calories 165; Fat Grams 1; Carbohydrate Grams 14; Protein Grams 25; Cholesterol mg 64; Sodium mg 137.

THE POINT SYSTEM: Calorie Points 2; Protein Points 3; Fat Grams 1; Sodium Points 6; Fiber Points 0; Carbohydrate Points 1; Cholesterol Points 6.

Apple Chicken Rolls

Serves: 4

Preparation Time: 1 hour

Equipment: French chef knife, cutting board, Kitchen Machine food cutter, medium skillet

¼	cup onions, chopped blade #3
1	cup (240 ml) unsweetened apple juice (or fresh juiced apples), divided
½	cup apple, chopped and peeled blade #3
½	cup soft rye breadcrumbs
2	tablespoons fresh parsley, minced
¼	teaspoon caraway seeds
4	4-ounce (115 g) boneless, skinless chicken breasts
2	tablespoons brandy
1	tablespoon cornstarch
	Apple slices for garnish (optional)

Preheat the medium skillet over medium heat; add onions, stirring dry-sauté 3-5 minutes until tender. Remove from heat and add 2-tablespoons apple juice, chopped apple, breadcrumbs, parsley and caraway seeds. Mix well, cover, close vent, and set aside.

Using a mallet, flatten to ¼-inch (75 mm) thickness. Divide breadcrumb mixture evenly between flattened chicken breasts, spoon mixture into center, and roll breasts lengthwise, tucking ends under. Secure with toothpicks. Clean skillet.

Preheat medium skillet over medium-high heat, about 3 minutes. Test the surface with a few water droplets. If the droplets bead up and dance across the surface, the pan is hot enough to brown the chicken and seal in juices. Place the chicken in the pan uncovered; it will stick at first. When the chicken loosens, turn gently and continue until brown on all sides. About 15 minutes.

Add 2 tablespoons apple juice and brandy cover, close vent, reduce to low-heat, and simmer 15 minutes. Transfer chicken to cutting board to rest.

Increase heat to medium, deglaze skillet with remaining apple juice, add cornstarch to pan juices in skillet, stir until mixture begins to thicken, remove from heat.

To serve, slice Apple Chicken Rolls to showoff spiral apple filling. Top with pan juices and garnish with sliced fresh apples.

NUTRITIONAL BREAKDOWN PER SERVING: Calories 391; Fat Grams 7; Carbohydrate Grams 20; Protein Grams 55; Cholesterol mg 146; Sodium mg 235.

THE POINT SYSTEM: Calorie Points 5; Protein Points 7; Fat Grams 7; Sodium Points 10; Fiber Points 0; Carbohydrate Points 1; Cholesterol Points 15.

Fish & Seafood...

Orange Roughly á la Asparagus

Serves: 8
Preparation Time: 25 minutes
Equipment: French chef knife, cutting board, 13-inch chef pan

I	pound (460 g) fresh asparagus spears cut into 1-inch (2.5 cm) pieces
I	2 ounce (60 g) jar pimientos, drained and diced
2	tablespoons fresh squeezed lemon juice
¼	teaspoon dried whole thyme (or fresh)
¼	teaspoon garlic powder or fresh, minced and crushed into a paste
¼	teaspoon fresh ground black pepper
3	pounds (1.4 kg) orange roughy fillets
2	tablespoons sliced almonds, toasted

In a mixing bowl, combine asparagus with pimiento, lemon juice, thyme, garlic powder and fresh grated pepper (optional). Set aside.

Arrange fillets in cool 13-inch (33 cm) chef pan, spoon asparagus mixture over fillets. Cover, close vent, and cook over medium-low heat 15-20 minutes, until fish flakes easily when tested with fork.

To serve, top with sliced almonds.

NUTRITIONAL BREAKDOWN PER SERVING: Calories 149; Fat Grams 2; Carbohydrate Grams 2; Protein Grams 29; Cholesterol mg 35; Sodium mg 178.

THE POINT SYSTEM: Calorie Points 2; Protein Points 4; Fat Grams 2; Sodium Points 8; Fiber Points 1; Carbohydrate Points 0; Cholesterol Points 4.

Scallops with Chives and Peppers

Serves: 4
Preparation Time: 15 minutes
Equipment: French chef knife, cutting board, large skillet

½   tablespoon olive oil
1   tablespoon unsalted butter, or low-calorie margarine
1   hot chili pepper, seeded and chopped (optional), or dried
½   red bell pepper, chopped
¾   pounds (360 g) fresh bay scallops
3   tablespoons fresh chives, chopped
     Pinch ground cloves or cinnamon

Preheat large skillet over medium-high heat, add olive oil and butter and bring to temperature. Add chili pepper, red pepper and sauté 2-3 minutes. Add scallops and sauté just long enough to heat through, about 2 minutes. Stir in chives, cloves and cinnamon. Sauté about 30 seconds more.

Serve over pasta or rice.

NUTRITIONAL BREAKDOWN PER SERVING: Calories 138; Fat Grams 5; Carbohydrate Grams 4; Protein Grams 21; Cholesterol mg 45; Sodium mg 261.

THE POINT SYSTEM: Calorie Points 2; Protein Points 3; Fat Grams 5; Sodium Points 11; Fiber Points 1; Carbohydrate Points ½; Cholesterol Points 5.

Spinach Fish Rolls

Serves: 6
Preparation Time: 40 minutes
Equipment: French chef knife, cutting board, Kitchen Machine food cutter,
medium stainless mixing bowl, large skillet

½	bag frozen spinach, chopped
½	cup feta cheese
½	cup low fat cottage cheese
2	teaspoons fresh grated lemon zest, blade #1
I	egg or 2 egg whites
3	gloves garlic, minced fine
I	teaspoon fresh oregano, minced fine (or dried)
6	thin fish fillets (sole)
I	small lemon, thinly sliced
I	tablespoon parsley, chopped

Drain excess water from spinach and cheese. In a mixing bowl, combine spinach, feta cheese, cottage cheese, lemon zest, egg, garlic and oregano. Mix well.

Place ¼ of spinach/cheese mixture in center of each fish fillet. Starting with the narrow end of the fillet, roll fillet over filling. Place seam-side down in large skillet, cover, close vent, and cook over medium-low heat for 30 minutes.

To serve, place on individual serving plates, garnish with lemon slice, and top with fresh chopped parsley.

NUTRITIONAL BREAKDOWN PER SERVING: Calories 257; Fat Grams 6; Carbohydrate Grams 10; Protein Grams 40; Cholesterol mg 104; Sodium mg 518.

THE POINT SYSTEM: Calorie Points 3½; Protein Points 5; Fat Grams 6; Sodium Points 23; Fiber Points 1; Carbohydrate Points ½; Cholesterol Points 10.

Italian Fish Rolls

Serves: 8
Preparation Time: 40 minutes
Equipment: French chef knife, cutting board, Kitchen Machine food cutter,
1-quart saucepan, medium stainless mixing bowl, large skillet

1	9 ounce (260 g) bag frozen French-style green beans
2	tablespoons onion, chopped blade #3
1	8 ounce (230 g) can tomato sauce or 1 cup homemade spaghetti sauce
¼	teaspoon fresh oregano, chopped or dried
¼	teaspoon fresh basil leaves, chopped
¼	teaspoon garlic, minced find, or powder
1	tablespoon Parmesan cheese, grated blade #1
8	flounder fillets without skin
1	tablespoon fresh basil, chopped

Place green beans and onions in 1-quart (1.5 L) saucepan, cover, close vent, and cook over medium heat 5 minutes; reduce heat to low for an additional 5 minutes. Remove from heat and set aside.

In the mixing bowl, combine tomato sauce, oregano, basil, garlic and Parmesan cheese.

Place one-eighth of bean mixture in the middle of each fillet. Starting at the narrow end, roll fillet over the filling. Place seam-side down in large skillet, and pour tomato sauce mixture over the top of fish rolls. Cover, close vent, and cook at medium-low heat 20-25 minutes.

To serve, remove fish fillets to individual serving plates, spoon sauce over fillets, and top with chopped basil.

NUTRITIONAL BREAKDOWN PER SERVING: Calories 260; Fat Grams 3; Carbohydrate Grams 4; Protein Grams 51; Cholesterol mg 96; Sodium mg 297.

THE POINT SYSTEM: Calorie Points 3½; Protein Points 6; Fat Grams 3; Sodium Points 13; Fiber Points 0; Carbohydrate Points ½; Cholesterol Points 9½.

Catfish Barbecue

Serves: 6
Preparation Time: 50 minutes
Equipment: French chef knife, cutting board, large skillet.

½	cup (120 ml) reduced calorie ketchup or barbecue sauce
1	tablespoon fresh squeezed lemon juice
1	teaspoon brown sugar
2	teaspoons vegetables oil
1	teaspoon low-sodium Worcestershire sauce
½	teaspoon dried whole marjoram
¼	teaspoon garlic powder
¼	teaspoon ground red pepper
6	4 ounce (120 g) farm-raised catfish fillets

In the mixing bowl combine ketchup, lemon juice, sugar, vegetable oil, Worcestershire sauce, marjoram, garlic powder and red pepper. Mix well.

Arrange fillets in large skillet and spoon ketchup mixture over fillets; cover and marinate in refrigerator 30 minutes to 1 hour, turning once.

Place 13-inch chef pan over medium heat, and bring to a simmer. Cover, close vent, and reduce the heat to low. Cook 15 minutes or until fish flakes easily when tested with a fork.

To serve, remove Catfish Fillets to individual serving plates and drizzle with sauce.

NUTRITIONAL BREAKDOWN PER SERVING: Calories 239; Fat Grams 14; Carbohydrate Grams 3; Protein Grams 25; Cholesterol mg 74; Sodium mg 193.

THE POINT SYSTEM: Calorie Points 3; Protein Points 3; Fat Grams 14; Sodium Points 8; Fiber Points 0; Carbohydrate Points 0; Cholesterol Points 7.

Shrimp, Scallop Jambalaya

Serves: 8
Preparation Time: 40 minutes
Equipment: French chef knife, cutting Board, Kitchen Machine food cutter, large skillet

1	medium onion, halved, peeled and chopped blade #3
1	large green pepper, seeded and chopped
½	cup celery, sliced blade #4 or waffle sliced blade #5
1	clove garlic, minced
1	32 ounce (290 g) can stewed tomatoes
1	cup (240 ml) water
1	cup long grain or brown rice, uncooked
1	bay leaf
½	teaspoon thyme, dried or fresh chopped
1	teaspoon basil, dried or fresh chopped
¼	teaspoon ground red pepper
1	pound fresh shrimp, or 12 ounce (340 g) package frozen shrimp, thawed
½	pound (230 g) bay scallops
2	tablespoons parsley or cilantro, chopped

In the large skillet, dry sauté onions, green pepper, celery and garlic over medium heat, about 10 minutes or until tender. Stir occasionally.

Add stewed tomatoes, water, rice, bay leaf, dried thyme, basil and red pepper. Mix well, cover, close vent, and simmer over medium-low heat 20-25 minutes. Add shrimp and scallops, cover and cook another 5-10 minutes or until rice is cooked through.

To serve, spoon Jambalaya into individual serving bowls, top with chopped parsley or cilantro.

NUTRITIONAL BREAKDOWN PER SERVING: Calories 175; Fat Grams 1; Carbohydrate Grams 24; Protein Grams 18; Cholesterol mg 79; Sodium mg 783.

THE POINT SYSTEM: Calorie Points 2½; Protein Points 2; Fat Grams 1; Sodium Points 34; Fiber Points 2; Carbohydrate Points 1½; Cholesterol Points 8.

Steamed Mussels

Serves: 8
Preparation Time: 40 minutes
Equipment: French chef knife, cutting board, 6-quart stockpot

1	teaspoon olive oil
2	medium onions, minced fine
4	cloves garlic, minced fine
2	cups (480 ml) red wine
4	dozen mussels*

In the 6-quart stockpot, sauté onions and garlic in olive oil over medium heat until tender, add wine and bring to a simmer. Add mussels, cover, open vent, and reduce heat to medium-low for 5-7 minutes or until mussels open.

To serve, spoon into individual soup bowls, top with wine sauce and serve with Garlic Bread recipe page 179.

Mussels* need to breath; remove from bag as soon as possible and submerge in fresh water. To clean mussels prior to cooking, soak in cold water with 4 tablespoons of cornstarch for 30 minutes. Scrape off beards, rinse, and soak again in fresh cold water. Discard any mussels that open before cooking. Do not eat mussels that do not open after cooking.

NUTRITIONAL BREAKDOWN PER SERVING: Calories 190; Fat Grams 4; Carbohydrate Grams 10; Protein Grams 17; Cholesterol mg 63; Sodium mg 364.

THE POINT SYSTEM: Calorie Points 3; Protein Points 2; Fat Grams 4; Sodium Points 16; Fiber Points ½; Carbohydrate Points 1; Cholesterol Points 6.

Mussels in Tomato Broth

Variation, use white wine instead of red wine, and add:

1	32 ounce (920 g) can plum tomatoes, chopped or crushed
1	cup parsley leaves, chopped
2	teaspoons dried oregano
1-2	tablespoons, hot crushed red pepper seeds (optional)

Simmer 15 minutes before adding mussels.

Nutritional breakdowns not included for this variation.

Thai Red Curry Shrimp and Pineapple

Serves: 8
Preparation Time: 20 minutes
Equipment: French chef knife, cutting Board, Kitchen Machine food cutter, large skillet

2	teaspoon vegetable oil or sesame seed oil
3	tablespoons red curry paste
1½	pounds (700 g) fresh shrimp, peeled, deveined, drained and dried
I	whole fresh pineapple, peeled and cubed
I	cup (240 ml) coconut milk, unsweetened
2	tablespoons raw sugar
½	teaspoon ground fennel seed
I	teaspoon turmeric
I	tablespoon fresh lime zest, grated blade #1
¼	cup (60 ml) low sodium soy sauce

Preheat vegetable oil in large skillet over medium-high heat until hot. Add red curry paste stirring to separate paste. Add shrimp, stir-fry about 3 minutes. Add pineapple and remaining ingredients, simmer 5-6 minutes.

Serve over prepared jasmine rice, garnish with cilantro and top with roasted peanuts.

NUTRITIONAL BREAKDOWN PER SERVING: Calories 187; Fat Grams 9; Carbohydrate Grams 14; Protein Grams 15; Cholesterol mg 102; Sodium mg 800.

THE POINT SYSTEM: Calorie Points 2½; Protein Points 2; Fat Grams 9; Sodium Points 35; Fiber Points I; Carbohydrate Points I; Cholesterol Points 10.

Paella

Serves: 16
Preparation Time: 45 minutes
Equipment: French chef knife, cutting board, Kitchen Machine food cutter, 13-inch chef pan

2	tablespoons olive oil
2	pounds (1 kg) chicken wings, trim wingtips, cut in half at joint
1	pound (460 g) chorizo
¼	pound (120 g) lean pork, cubed
¼	pound (120 g) precooked ham, cubed
3	onions, halved peeled and chopped blade #3
2	green peppers, chopped
4	cloves garlic, minced
3	fresh tomatoes, quartered and seeded
1	teaspoon oregano
5	cups (1.25 L) water
½	teaspoon sea salt or kosher salt
¼	teaspoon fresh ground pepper
2	cups uncooked rice
¼	teaspoon saffron
1	pound (460 g) cooked shrimp
½	pound (230 g) cooked lobster, cubed
1	10 ounce (300 g) package frozen peas
1	32 ounce (920 g) can artichoke hearts
16	clams or mussels
1	4 ounce (120 g) can pimentos, sliced

Preheat 13-inch chef pan over medium-high heat, about 2-3 minutes. Add the oil and bring to temperature, add chicken, chorizo, pork, ham, and sauté until browned. Add onions, peppers and garlic, sauté 3-5 minutes until tender. Add tomatoes and oregano, water, salt, pepper, rice and saffron. Mix well, cover, open vent, and reduce to medium heat, simmer 15 minutes. Add shrimp, lobster, peas, artichokes, pimentos and mussels (clams). Cover, close vent, reduce to low heat, cook 15-20 minutes, or until rice is cooked through and mussels have opened.

To serve, place chef pan on trivet and serve pan. Top with pimentos.

NUTRITIONAL BREAKDOWN PER SERVING: Calories 341; Fat Grams 16; Carbohydrate Grams 25; Protein Grams 26; Cholesterol mg 96; Sodium mg 656.

THE POINT SYSTEM: Calorie Points 4½; Protein Points 3; Fat Grams 16; Sodium Points 29; Fiber Points 3; Carbohydrate Points 1½; Cholesterol Points 10.

NOTE: in Spain and in Spanish communities worldwide there are hundreds of authentic Paella recipes, typically dictated by fresh ingredients available in the region. Olive oil, saffron, and rice are typically the common ingredient in all Paella recipes.

Shrimp Spring Rolls

Serves: 8
Preparation Time: 30 minutes
Equipment: French chef knife, cutting board, Kitchen Machine food cutter, large skillet,
medium stainless mixing bowl, stainless cookie sheet

8	Spring Roll wrappers (available frozen at Oriental and health food markets)
½	cup dried black mushrooms (shitake or wood ear) soaked in hot water, 10 minutes
3	tablespoons peanut oil
I	pound (460 g) shrimp, peeled, deveined, and chopped
3	shallots, minced
I	clove garlic, mince
I	teaspoon fresh ginger, grated blade #1
I	celery rib, minced
I	Serrano chili, minced
I	carrot, grated blade #1
½	pound (230 g) fresh bean sprouts
I	tablespoon soy sauce
I	teaspoon sesame oil
I	tablespoon sake or dry sherry
½	teaspoon 5-spice mix, see recipe page 204
2	teaspoons cornstarch
½	cup (120 ml) water
I	tablespoon cornstarch

Preheat large skillet or 13-inch chef pan over medium-high heat, add peanut oil and bring to temperature, add shrimp and sauté about 30 seconds. Add mushrooms and all vegetables, stir-fry 1-2 minutes, adding bean sprouts last.

In mixing bowl, combine soy sauce, sesame oil, sake, and 5-spice mix with 2 teaspoons cornstarch. Mix well and add to wok and toss to combine. Stir until mixture thickens (about 1 minute). Spread mixture onto cookie sheet to cool.

Mix together water and 1 tablespoon cornstarch to seal edges. Roll each wrapper, "Burrito" style, by placing approximately 2 tablespoons of filling one-third the way up the wrapper. Fold corners over filling forming a lightly packed log shaped roll. Fold side edges over and roll to end of wrapper. Seal edges with cornstarch, water mixture and finish rolling.

In the skillet, fry 2-4 spring rolls at a time, in 1-2 inches of peanut oil over medium-high heat, turning until golden brown on all sides. Drain on paper towels and serve.

NUTRITIONAL BREAKDOWN PER SERVING: Calories 117; Fat Grams 2; Carbohydrate Grams 9; Protein Grams 14; Cholesterol mg 85; Sodium mg 563.

THE POINT SYSTEM: Calorie Points 2; Protein Points 2; Fat Grams 2; Sodium Points 24; Fiber Points 1; Carbohydrate Points ½; Cholesterol Points 8.

Soy Dipping Sauce

Yields: 2 cups
Preparation Time: 10 minutes
Equipment: French chef knife, Cutting Board, small stainless mixing bowl

½   cup (120 ml) water
½   cup (120 ml) white distiller vinegar or rice vinegar
½   cup (120 ml) soy sauce
½   cup sugar
1   teaspoon chili paste
2   teaspoons garlic, minced fine

In the mixing bowl, combine all ingredients. Serve with Spring Rolls and Oriental recipes.

NUTRITIONAL BREAKDOWN PER SERVING: Calories 71; Fat Grams 0; Carbohydrate Grams 17; Protein Grams 2; Cholesterol mg 0; Sodium mg 538.

THE POINT SYSTEM: Calorie Points 1; Protein Points 1; Fat Grams 0; Sodium Points 23; Fiber Points 0; Carbohydrate Points 1; Cholesterol Points 0.

Poached Salmon

Serves: 6
Preparation Time: 35 minutes
Equipment: French chef knife, cutting board, Kitchen Machine food cutter, large skillet

4	cups (1 L) water
½	cup onion, chopped blade #3
½	cup carrots, sliced blade #4 or waffle sliced blade #5
½	cup celery, sliced blade #4
2	cloves garlic, minced
6	pepper corns
4	allspice, whole
1	teaspoon Bouquet Garni, see recipe page 205
2	tablespoon fresh squeezed lemon juice
1	pound (460 g) salmon fillet
½	fresh lemon, sliced thin
3-4	sprigs fresh thyme

In the large skillet, combine all ingredients except salmon. Bring to a simmer over medium-high heat, and then reduce to medium-low heat for 5 minutes. Place fillet in skillet and continue to simmer, approximately 15 minutes.

To serve, remove fillet with spatula to a serving platter, garnish with lemon slices, top with fresh thyme, and serve with fresh vegetables or rice.

NUTRITIONAL BREAKDOWN PER SERVING: Calories 108; Fat Grams 3; Carbohydrate Grams 5; Protein Grams 16; Cholesterol mg 39; Sodium mg 73.

THE POINT SYSTEM: Calorie Points 1½; Protein Points 2; Fat Grams 3; Sodium Points 3; Fiber Points ½; Carbohydrate Points ½; Cholesterol Points 4.

Sweet & Sour Tuna

Serves: 8
Preparation Time: 15 minutes
Equipment: French chef knife, cutting board, Kitchen Machine food cutter, 13-inch chef pan

6	slices canned pineapple
1	tablespoon olive oil
½	cup (160 ml) pineapple juice
2	green bell peppers cut into 1-inch (2.5 cm) strips
2	tablespoons cornstarch
2	teaspoons low sodium soy sauce
2	tablespoons white distilled or rice vinegar
3	tablespoons raw sugar
1	cup (240 ml) low sodium chicken broth, or homemade chicken stock
1	14 ounce (400 g) can water-packed tuna or 1 pound fresh tuna
4-6	cups cooked rice or crisp noodles

In the 13-inch (33 cm) chef pan, sauté pineapple in olive oil for 5 minutes over medium heat to caramelize. Add ¼ cup pineapple juice and green pepper. Cover, open vent, and simmer 10 minutes.

Mix cornstarch with remaining pineapple juice, add to pan with soy sauce, vinegar, sugar and chicken broth. Stir until mixture thickens. Add tuna, cover, and cook about 5 minutes. If using fresh tuna, cook 10-12 minutes or until tuna flakes easily with a fork.

To serve, place crisp Chinese noodles or rice on individual serving plates, and spoon tuna mixture and sauce, top with a small dollop of Chinese hot mustard, if desired.

NUTRITIONAL BREAKDOWN PER SERVING: Calories 206; Fat Grams 3; Carbohydrate Grams 30; Protein Grams 15; Cholesterol mg 15; Sodium mg 224.

THE POINT SYSTEM: Calorie Points 2 ½; Protein Points 2; Fat Grams 3; Sodium Points 10; Fiber Points 0; Carbohydrate Points 2; Cholesterol Points 1.

Seafood Filé Gumbo

Serves: 6
Preparation Time: 50 minutes
Equipment: French chef knife, cutting board, Kitchen Machine food cutter,
3-quart saucepan, 6-quart stockpot

5	cups (1.25 L) water
1	teaspoon Old Bay seasoning
6	crayfish, fresh or cooked
½	pound (230 g) pork shoulder cut in 1½" cubed
2	tablespoons unsalted butter or low calorie margarine
1	onion, sliced
1	green pepper, seeded and sliced
2	cloves garlic, minced
3	tablespoons flour
½	teaspoon thyme, fresh or dried
1	bay leaf
2	tablespoons fresh parsley, chopped
½	teaspoon Worcestershire sauce
12	oysters, fresh or frozen
1	pound (460 g) fresh shrimp, peeled and deveined
8	plum tomatoes, seeded and chopped (peeled if time permits)
2	cups sliced okra, blade #4 or waffle slice blade #5
2	tablespoons filé powder

In the 3-quart (3 L utensil) saucepan, bring water to a boil over medium-high heat. Add Old Bay and crayfish; simmer about 8-10 minutes.

Preheat the 6-quart stockpot over medium-high heat, about 3 minutes. Place the pork in the pan; it will stick at first while browning. Cover the pan and open the vent. When the pork loosens, about 3-5 minutes, turn to brown on all sides. Remove to a platter. To the 6-quart Stockpot, add butter, onion, pepper and garlic, and sauté until tender, about 3-4 minutes. To make a Roux, sprinkle in flour a little bit at a time, and stir constantly until flour turns a pale golden brown. Gradually add strained crayfish stock and continue to stir until crayfish stock and onion, pepper, roux is completely incorporated. Add thyme, bay leaf, parsley, Worcestershire sauce, oysters, shrimp, crayfish, tomatoes and reserved pork, and bring to a simmer. Stir in okra and filé powder. Continue to cook until Gumbo thickens.

To serve, spoon Gumbo into individual serving bowls, or spoon Gumbo over cooked rice.

NUTRITIONAL BREAKDOWN PER SERVING: Calories 432; Fat Grams 8; Carbohydrate Grams 52; Protein Grams 39; Cholesterol mg 59; Sodium mg 732.

THE POINT SYSTEM: Calorie Points 6; Protein Points 5; Fat Grams 8; Sodium Points 32; Fiber Points 1; Carbohydrate Points 3 ½; Cholesterol Points 16.

Singapore Fish

Serves: 6
Preparation Time: 30 minutes
Equipment: French Chef Knife, cutting board, medium stainless Mixing Bowl,
13-inch chef pan, small mixing bowl

I	pound (460 g) halibut fillets*, skin removed, cut into 2-inch cubes
I	egg white
I	tablespoon cornstarch
2	teaspoons white wine or rice wine
	Peanut oil for frying
I	large onion cut in ½-inch wedges
I	tablespoon curry powder
2	teaspoons raw sugar (optional)
I	20 ounce (750 g) can pineapple chunks (reserve juice) or fresh
I	11 ounce (310 g) can mandarin oranges (reserve juice)
I	8 ounce (230 g) can water chestnuts, drained
I	tablespoon cornstarch mixed well with juice of
I	fresh lime

In the medium mixing bowl, whisk egg white to a slight froth, add cornstarch, wine, and mix well. Place halibut in mixture to coat.

Heat oil in 13-inch (33 cm) chef pan over medium-high heat, add a few pieces of halibut at a time and fry all sides until golden brown. With a slotted spoon, remove halibut to paper towel to drain. Continue until all fish

In the small mixing bowl, combine cornstarch and lime juice, mix well.

Remove oil from chef pan, add onion, and stir-fry 1-2 minutes. Add curry powder, stir-fry 1-2 minutes. Add reserved juices; bring to a simmer over medium heat.

Add lime and cornstarch mixture, stir into boiling juices. Add sugar, pineapple, orange, water chestnuts, and fried fish, stir to coat. Heat through 1 minute, and serve immediately.

*Chicken may be substituted for halibut.

NUTRITIONAL BREAKDOWN PER SERVING: Calories 250; Fat Grams 11; Carbohydrate Grams 21; Protein Grams 17; Cholesterol mg 24; Sodium mg 58.

THE POINT SYSTEM: Calorie Points 3 ½; Protein Points 2; Fat Grams 11; Sodium Points 2 ½; Fiber Points 1; Carbohydrate Points 1 ½; Cholesterol Points 2.

Eggs & Cheese...

Strawberry Cheese Blintzes

Yields: 12, Serves: 6
Preparation Time: 20 minutes
Equipment: Kitchen Machine food cutter, 3-quart stainless mixing bowl, 13-inch chef pan

1½	cups non-fat cottage cheese
½	cup light cream cheese
2	egg whites, whisked to a light froth
2	tablespoons honey
1	teaspoon lemon zest, grated blade #1
½	teaspoon vanilla
12	crêpes (basic recipe below)
½	cup Frozen Strawberry Jam thawed, see recipe page 146
¼	cup non-fat sour cream

In the 3-quart mixing bowl, combine cottage cheese, cream cheese, frothed egg whites, honey, lemon zest and vanilla. Spoon 3 tablespoons cheese mixture into the center of each crêpe, fold right over left over filling forming a square, then roll to form blintz. To warm, place blintzes seam side down in 13-inch chef pan, cover, close vent, and warm over low heat for 10 minutes.

To serve, top with strawberry Jam, a dollop of sour cream, garnish with mint leaves.

Basic Crêpes

Yields: 6 portions
Preparation Time: 30 minutes
Equipment: 2-quart stainless mixing bowl, 10-inch chef pan

1	cup sifted flour
½	teaspoon salt
3	eggs well beaten
1	cup (240 ml) milk
	Cooking spray

Combine flour, salt, eggs, milk, and whisk. Spray 8-inch chef pan with cooking spray, heat over medium-high 2-3 minutes. Pour 2 tablespoons batter into pan, lift pan and tilt, side to side to coat evenly, return to heat. Cook until lightly browned, and slide crêpe onto plate. Repeat process.

NUTRITIONAL BREAKDOWN PER SERVING: Calories 132; Fat Grams 4; Carbohydrate Grams 17; Protein Grams 8; Cholesterol mg 4; Sodium mg 290.

THE POINT SYSTEM: Calorie Points 2; Protein Points 1; Fat Grams 4; Sodium Points 13; Fiber Points 0; Carbohydrate Points 1; Cholesterol Points 0.

Spinach & Cheese Jumbo Shells

Serves: 10

Preparation Time: 50 minutes

Equipment: Kitchen Machine food cutter, 6½ quart 'tall' stockpot,
6-quart pasta/steamer basket, 3-quart stainless mixing bowl

1   12 ounce (340 g) box jumbo shells

FILLING

2	pounds (1 kg) low-fat ricotta cheese
1	cup mozzarella cheese, shredded blade #3
½	cup Romano cheese, grated blade #1
½	teaspoon fresh grated black pepper
3	eggs, whisked well before adding, or 6 egg whites
1	10 ounce (300 g) package frozen chopped spinach, thawed and drained
3	cup Marinara Sauce*
2	tablespoons Parmesan cheese, grated blade #1
2	teaspoons fresh parsley, chopped

With 6-quart pasta/steamer basket inserted into 6½-quart stockpot and bring 4 quarts of water to a boil over medium-high heat. Place shells in pasta/steamer insert, and cook only 8-10 minutes. Shells should still feel firm. Remove Pasta insert and rinse shells under cold water to stop cooking process. Set aside to drain.

In the mixing bowl combine ricotta and mozzarella cheese, pepper, eggs and spinach, mix well. Fill each shell with approximately 1 tablespoon filling. Cover the bottom of the (cold) 13-inch chef pan with 1 cup Marinara sauce and place stuffed shells seam-side up in the Pan. Cover the shells with the balance of the Marinara sauce. Cover, open vent, and cook over medium-low heat 20-25 minutes.

To serve, place in individual serving bowls, spoon sauce over, top with Parmesan cheese and garnish with chopped parsley.

Marinara sauce is not included in nutritional breakdown. See recipe page 155.

NUTRITIONAL BREAKDOWN PER SERVING: Calories 291; Fat Grams 10; Carbohydrate Grams 25; Protein Grams 23; Cholesterol mg 24; Sodium mg 704.

THE POINT SYSTEM: Calorie Points 4; Protein Points 3; Fat Grams 10; Sodium Points 31; Fiber Points 1; Carbohydrate Points 1½; Cholesterol Points 2.

Mardi-Gras Family Omelet

Serves: 10
Preparation Time: 30 minutes
Equipment: French Chef Knife, cutting board, Kitchen Machine food cutter, 10-inch chef pan,
13-inch chef pan, 3-quart stainless mixing bowl

½	pound (230 g) Italian sausage, removed from casing
1	tablespoon beef broth or homemade beef stock
½	green bell pepper, seeded and sliced
½	red bell pepper, seeded and sliced
½	yellow bell pepper, seeded and sliced
6	mushrooms, sliced blade #4 (to slice, lay mushrooms sideways in hopper)
8	eggs or equivalent egg substitute* (16 egg whites)
2	tablespoons skim milk
3	tablespoons unsalted butter
2	plum tomatoes, sliced
½	cup Monterey Jack cheese, shredded blade #2
½	cup cheddar cheese, shredded blade #2
¼	cup green onion, chopped

In the 10-inch chef pan, brown sausage over medium-high heat, drain sausage on paper towels.

In the 13-inch chef pan sauté peppers and mushrooms in beef broth over medium heat until softened, remove to side dish. Clean skillet to cook omelet.

In the 3-quart mixing bowl, beat eggs with milk.

Melt butter in 13-inch chef pan over medium heat, add beaten eggs, cover, open vent, and cook 10 minutes or until eggs are almost set.

To one side of the omelet, add peppers and mushrooms, tomatoes, and half the cheese. Using a flexible spatula, flip omelet over vegetables; top with remaining cheese. Cover, close the vent, reduce to low heat, and cook an additional 5 minutes to allow cheese to melt.

To serve, slide omelet onto serving platter, top with chopped green onions.

* Nutritional breakdown uses egg substitutes.

NUTRITIONAL BREAKDOWN PER SERVING: Calories 216; Fat Grams 15; Carbohydrate Grams 6; Protein Grams 13; Cholesterol mg 44; Sodium mg 631.

THE POINT SYSTEM: Calorie Points 3; Protein Points 2; Fat Grams 15; Sodium Points 27; Fiber Points 1; Carbohydrate Points ½; Cholesterol Points 4.

Egg Casserole

Serves: 12
Preparation Time: 1 hour 15 minutes
Equipment: French Chef Knife, cutting board, 13-inch chef pan, 5-quart stainless mixing bowl

1	pound (460 g) Italian sausage removed from casing or ground turkey,
2	teaspoons sage, add only when using turkey
6	slices bread, cubed with crust removed
2	cups (480 ml) skim milk
4	eggs, beaten or 8 egg whites
1	teaspoon prepared mustard
½	teaspoon sea salt or kosher salt (optional)
¼	pound (120 g) cheddar cheese, shredded blade #3
1	tablespoon fresh parsley, chopped

In the 13-inch (33 cm) chef pan or large skillet sauté sausage over medium heat until cooked through, and remove to paper towels to drain. Clean chef pan to cook casserole.

In the 5-quart mixing bowl, combine all ingredients.

Lightly coat 13-inch chef pan with cooking spray, pour casserole ingredients, cover, open the vent, and cook over medium heat for 15 minutes, reduce heat to low and continue cooking 30-40 minutes, or until casserole is cooked through and firm.

Variation, bake in preheated 350°F (180°C) oven 1 hour, removing the cover the last 15 minutes.

To serve, top with chopped parsley and serve from chef skillet.

Nutritional breakdown uses whole eggs.

NUTRITIONAL BREAKDOWN PER SERVING: Calories 175; Fat Grams 9; Carbohydrate Grams 9; Protein Grams 13; Cholesterol mg 159; Sodium mg 427.

THE POINT SYSTEM: Calorie Points 2½; Protein Points 2; Fat Grams 9; Sodium Points 18½; Fiber Points 0; Carbohydrate Points ½; Cholesterol Points 16.

Breakfast Burritos

Yields: 24 - Serves: 12
Preparation Time: 20 minutes
Equipment: large skillet, large stainless mixing bowl, 13-inch chef skillet

2	pounds (1 kg) Italian sausage, removed from casing
2	tablespoons chili powder
1	teaspoon cumin
1	tablespoon paprika
¼	cup (60 ml) skim milk
12	eggs or equivalent egg substitutes*
2	tablespoons unsalted butter or low calorie margarine
24	8-inch (20 cm) tortillas**
	Salsa recipe below

In the 13-inch chef skillet, over medium heat, sauté sausage with chili powder, cumin, paprika, and cook until browned. Clean chef pan to prepare eggs.

In the mixing bowl, whisk milk and eggs together to a froth.

In the 13-inch (33 cm) chef pan, melt butter over medium heat, and French scramble eggs with sausage mixture. Place 2 heaping tablespoons of egg, sausage mixture in individual tortilla shells and "burrito" roll. Add salsa to taste and serve immediately.

*Nutritional breakdown uses egg substitutes and includes salsa.

Salsa

Yields: 2 ½ cups
Preparation Time: 10 minutes
Equipment: Kitchen Machine food cutter, medium mixing bowl

4	Roma or plum tomatoes, seeded and chopped
¼	cup cilantro, chopped
½	cup white onion, peeled and chopped #2 blade
½	fresh lemon, juice of
	Salt & pepper to taste (optional)

In the 2-quart mixing bowl, combine ingredients, serve at room temperature

NUTRITIONAL BREAKDOWN PER SERVING: Calories 134; Fat Grams 18; Carbohydrate Grams 21; Protein Grams 15; Cholesterol mg 0; Sodium mg 299.

THE POINT SYSTEM: Calorie Points 2; Protein Points 2; Fat Grams 18; Sodium Points 13; Fiber Points 0; Carbohydrate Points 1½; Cholesterol Points 0.

Frozen Strawberry Jam

Serves: 16
Preparation Time: 20 minutes
Equipment: stainless mixing bowl, 2-quart saucepan

I   quart whole fresh strawberries
I   cup (240 ml) cherry juice concentrate
I   packet unflavored gelatin
I   teaspoon fresh squeezed lemon juice

Wash strawberries and remove stems, and mash with potato masher or fork, in the mixing bowl.

In the 2-quart (2 L) saucepan bring cherry juice to a boil over medium-high heat. Stir in gelatin, about 1 minute. Remove from heat and stir in strawberries and lemon juice.

For individual servings, pour into ice cube trays, when frozen, pop out of trays and place in large plastic bags and return to freezer.

NUTRITIONAL BREAKDOWN PER SERVING: Calories 19; Fat Grams 0; Carbohydrate Grams 4; Protein Grams I; Cholesterol mg 0; Sodium mg I.

THE POINT SYSTEM: Calorie Points 0; Protein Points 0; Fat Grams 0; Sodium Points 0; Fiber Points 0; Carbohydrate Points 0; Cholesterol Points 0.

Egg Fu Yung

Serves: 4
Preparation Time: 30 minutes
Equipment: I-quart saucepan, French chef knife, cutting board,
3-quart stainless mixing bowl, 8-inch chef pan, 7-inch chef pan

SAUCE

I	cup (240 ml) chicken broth or homemade chicken or beef stock
I	teaspoon ketchup
I	dash sesame oil
I	tablespoon soy sauce
I	tablespoon cornstarch
3	tablespoons water

EGGS

5	eggs or equivalent egg substitute*
I	tablespoon water
½	cup shredded cooked beef, pork, chicken or crab
I	tablespoon unsalted butter, vegetable oil or cooking spray
I	small onion, sliced thin or chopped
I	celery rib, finely chopped
2	ounces (60 g) bean sprouts
½	cup shredded cooked meat, poultry or fish
4	Chinese dried mushrooms, soaked in boiling water 5 minutes

For sauce, in the I-quart (I.5 L) saucepan, bring chicken stock, ketchup, sesame oil, and soy sauce to a simmer over medium heat. Combine cornstarch and water, mix and add to sauce, whisk until thickened. Remove from heat, cover to keep hot, and set aside.

In the 8-inch skillet, spray pan with cooking spray, sauté onion and celery over medium heat until tender but crisp, about 3-4 minutes. Set aside.

In the mixing bowl, whisk eggs and water lightly, stir in shredded meat, onion, celery and bean sprouts. Squeeze liquid from mushrooms, remove stems, cut caps into thin slices and add to egg mixture. Add the bean sprouts and onions, and mix well.

Spray the 7-inch or 8-inch chef pan (or both) with cooking spray or use a small amount of butter, place over medium heat, when hot, spoon in about one-quarter of egg mixture. Brown one side and turn gently, brown second side. Remove to platter, keep warm, and continue to cook additional egg fu yung servings.

*Nutritional breakdown uses egg substitute. To reduce sodium by 325mg omit soy sauce.

NUTRITIONAL BREAKDOWN PER SERVING: Calories 138; Fat Grams 5; Carbohydrate Grams 10; Protein Grams 13; Cholesterol mg 13; Sodium mg 1100.

THE POINT SYSTEM: Calorie Points 1½; Protein Points 1½; Fat Grams 5; Sodium Points 47; Fiber Points 0; Carbohydrate Points ½; Cholesterol Points 1.

Cheese Fondue

Serves: 4
Preparation Time: 30 minutes
Equipment: French chef knife, cutting board, Kitchen Machine food cutter,
2-quart saucepan, 5-quart stainless mixing bowl

2	cups (480 ml) dry white wine
1	tablespoon fresh squeezed lemon juice
1	pound (460 g) Gruyere cheese, shredded blade #3
1	pound (460 g) Fontina cheese, shredded blade #3
1	tablespoon arrowroot
2	ounces (60 ml) kirsch (optional)
1	pinch nutmeg
1	loaf French bread or whole wheat loaf, cubed
4	pears cut in wedges
4	apples cut in wedges

Combine wine and lemon juice in 2 quart Saucepan (2 L) and bring to a simmer over medium heat, and reduce to low. Gradually add cheese mixture to wine, stirring constantly. When cheeses are melted, stir in arrowroot and kirsch.

To serve, sprinkle with nutmeg. Place French bread, apples and pears at the end of skewer forks, dip in hot cheese mixture, enjoy.

NUTRITIONAL BREAKDOWN PER SERVING: Calories 471; Fat Grams 26; Carbohydrate Grams 31; Protein Grams 24; Cholesterol mg 85; Sodium mg 583.

THE POINT SYSTEM: Calorie Points 6½; Protein Points 3; Fat Grams 26; Sodium Points 25; Fiber Points 1; Carbohydrate Points2; Cholesterol Points 8½.

Vegetables...

Potato Salad

Serves: 20
Preparation Time: 1 hour
Equipment: French chef knife, cutting board, Kitchen Machine food cutter

10	medium red potatoes, cooked waterless and cubed
½	cup celery, chopped
½	cup red onion, chopped blade #3
1	cup sour cream or low-fat plain yogurt
½	cup low-fat mayonnaise
½	teaspoon onion powder
½	teaspoon garlic powder
½	teaspoon pepper
½	teaspoon celery salt
2	eggs hard cooked, quartered (see recipe page 31)
1	firm tomato, quartered
¼	cup green onions, chopped

In a large bowl combine potatoes with celery, onion, sour cream or yogurt, mayonnaise, onion and garlic powder, pepper and celery salt, and toss well. Cover and refrigerate until ready to serve.

To serve, top with hard cooked eggs and tomatoes, sprinkle with chopped green onions.

NUTRIONAL BREAKDOWN PER SERVING: Calories 32; Fat Grams 0; Carbohydrate Grams 7; Protein Grams 1; Cholesterol mg 0; Sodium mg 124.

THE POINT SYSTEM: Calorie Points ½; Protein Points 0; Fat Grams 0; Sodium Points 5; Fiber Points 0; Carbohydrate Points ½; Cholesterol Points 0.

Spicy Carrots

Serves: 6
Preparation Time: 20 minutes
Equipment: French chef knife, cutting board, Kitchen Machine food cutter, large skillet

2	teaspoons safflower
1	tablespoon garlic, minced
1	tablespoon ginger, grated blade #1
½	teaspoon crushed red pepper
1½	pounds (700 g) carrots, scrubbed well and cut in diagonal pieces
⅔	cups (160 ml) chicken broth or homemade chicken stock
3	tablespoons soy sauce
2	tablespoons apple cider vinegar
2	teaspoons raw sugar
1	tablespoon cornstarch
2	tablespoon water

Preheat oil in the large skillet over medium-high heat. Add garlic, ginger, and red pepper, stir well. Add carrots, chicken stock, soy sauce, cider vinegar, sugar, and stir. Bring to a simmer, cover (close vent) and reduce the heat to low. Cook about 10-12 minutes or until carrots are tender.

Combine cornstarch and water, and stir until smooth. Stir into spicy carrots and cook 1-2 minutes until slightly thickened.

NUTRITIONAL BREAKDOWN PER SERVING: Calories 84; Fat Grams 2; Carbohydrate Grams 16; Protein Grams 2; Cholesterol mg 0; Sodium mg 641 (440 with homemade chicken stock).

THE POINT SYSTEM: Calorie Points 1; Protein Points 0; Fat Grams 2; Sodium Points 28 (18 with homemade chicken stock); Fiber Points 1; Carbohydrate Points 1; Cholesterol Points 0.

Vegetable Stir Fry

Serves: 4
Preparation Time: 25 minutes
Equipment: French chef knife, cutting board, Kitchen Machine food cutter, 11-inch wok

2	teaspoons sesame oil
1	cup broccoli florets cut into 1-inch (2.5 cm) pieces
1	large carrot, sliced blade #4
1	zucchini, sliced blade #4 or julienned blade #3
1	red onion, quartered and julienned blade #2
1	tablespoon water
½	cup fresh mushrooms, sliced blade #4 (to slice, place sideways in hopper)
¼	teaspoon fresh dill, chopped
4	cherry tomatoes, halved

Heat oil in wok or large skillet over medium-high heat; add broccoli, carrots, zucchini and onion. Stir-fry 4-5 minutes. Add water, cover (close vent) reduces heat to medium-low and cook 5-7 minutes. Stir in dill, add mushroom, tomatoes, recover and cook 5 minutes or until vegetables are tender.

NUTRITIONAL BREAKDOWN PER SERVING: Calories 70; Fat Grams 3; Carbohydrate Grams 11; Protein Grams 2; Cholesterol mg 0; Sodium mg 159.

THE POINT SYSTEM: Calorie Points 1; Protein Points 0; Fat Grams 3; Sodium Points 7; Fiber Points 1; Carbohydrate Points ½; Cholesterol Points 0.

Asparagus Mushroom Sauté

Serves: 4
Preparation Time: 15 minutes
Equipment: French chef knife, cutting board, Kitchen Machine food cutter, large skillet

2	tablespoons chicken broth or homemade chicken stock
¼	pound (120 g) fresh mushrooms, sliced blade #4 (to slice, sideways in hopper)
¼	cup red bell pepper, diced
¼	onion, peeled and julienned blade #2
1	16 ounce (460 g) can asparagus cuts and tips drained or 1 pound fresh
¼	cup (60 ml) dry white wine
1	teaspoon cornstarch
1	teaspoon fresh tarragon leaves, chopped
1	teaspoon fresh lemon zest, grated blade #1
1	teaspoon fresh squeezed lemon juice

Heat chicken broth in large skillet over medium-high heat; add mushrooms, red pepper and onion, sauté about 2 minutes or until tender. Add asparagus and sauté 1-2 minutes. Combine wine and cornstarch; stir to dissolve. Add remaining ingredients stir-fry about 1 minute until sauce simmers and thickens.

To serve, top with chopped tarragon and lemon zest, drizzle lemon juice and serve.

NUTRITIONAL BREAKDOWN PER SERVING: Calories 57; Fat Grams 1; Carbohydrate Grams 6; Protein Grams 4; Cholesterol mg 0; Sodium mg 42.

THE POINT SYSTEM: Calorie Points ½; Protein Points ½; Fat Grams 1; Sodium Points 2; Fiber Points 1; Carbohydrate Points ½; Cholesterol Points 0.

Eggplant Parmigiana

Serves: 8
Preparation Time: 1 hour
Equipment: French chef knife, cutting board, Kitchen Machine food cutter,
13-inch chef pan, large skillet

3	medium eggplants, sliced into ½-inch rings
3	cups (720 ml) Marinara sauce, see page 155
2	cups mushrooms, shredded blade #2 (optional)
3	cups mozzarella cheese, shredded blade #3
¼	cup Romano cheese, grated blade #1
	Fresh basil, whole or chopped

Slice eggplants, sprinkle with salt, and place on paper towel or dish towel in between each ring, creating a stack of eggplant. Place something heavy, like a large skillet or a heavy book on top of stack of eggplant rings. By salting and pressing, bitterness, if any, is removed. Press about 20-30 minutes, rinse and pat dry.

Preheat the 13-inch (33 cm) chef pan over medium heat, add olive oil and bring to temperature. Add enough eggplant rings to fill pan, fry both sides until golden brown and remove to paper towels to drain.

Cover the bottom of the large skillet with a layer of Marinara sauce, place one layer of eggplant across the bottom, layer with a mixture of mushrooms, and mozzarella cheese, top with a layer of Marinara sauce, then repeat the process. Top layer, mozzarella and sprinkle with Romano cheese. Cover, close the vent, and cook over medium-low heat for 30 minutes.

To serve, remove from heat and let stand 10-15 minutes, with s serrated knife, slice into 8 individual servings. Top with fresh basil and serve.

NUTRITIONAL BREAKDOWN PER SERVING: Calories 226; Fat Grams 13; Carbohydrate Grams 11; Protein Grams 18; Cholesterol mg 39; Sodium mg 906.

THE POINT SYSTEM: Calorie Points 3; Protein Points 2; Fat Grams 13; Sodium Points 39; Fiber Points 1; Carbohydrate Points ½; Cholesterol Points 4.

Marinara Sauce

Serves: 12 – 1 cup servings
Yields: 2-quarts (2 L)
Equipment: French chef knife, cutting board, Kitchen Machine food cutter, 4-quart stockpot

2	tablespoons olive oil
½	cup onion, chopped blade #3
1	12 ounce can (345 g) tomato paste
½	cup (120 ml) red wine
5	cups (1.25 L) water
1	tablespoon dried basil, or fresh, chopped
1	tablespoon oregano dried, or fresh, chopped
2	tablespoons fresh parsley, chopped
1	14.5 ounces (435 g) can diced tomatoes,
	or 1¼ pounds plum tomatoes, peeled, seeded and diced

In the 4-quart (4 L) stockpot sauté onion in olive oil over medium heat until tender, about 5 minutes. Add tomato paste and fry until tomato paste turns Indian red. Tomato paste will leave a sugar residue on bottom of pan, stir continuously to prevent from sticking or burning. Deglaze pan with wine and cook down until tomato wine mixture thickens and alcohol is cooked off.

Add water, spices and tomatoes, mix well and simmer uncovered 45 to 1 hour or until reduced by about one-third.

To serve, use in preparation of Eggplant Parmigiana, page 154, or Spinach Jumbo Shells page 142.

NUTRITIONAL BREAKDOWN PER SERVING: Calories 73; Fat Grams 3; Carbohydrate Grams 9; Protein Grams 1; Cholesterol mg 0; Sodium mg 330.

THE POINT SYSTEM: Calorie Points 1; Protein Points 0; Fat Grams 3; Sodium Points 14; Fiber Points 0; Carbohydrate Points ½; Cholesterol Points 0.

Rosemary Potatoes

Serves: 8

Preparation Time: 1 hour 10 minutes

Equipment: French chef knife, cutting board, Kitchen Machine food cutter, 4-quart stockpot

1	tablespoon olive oil
1	tablespoon unsalted butter
1	tablespoon fresh rosemary, chopped
1	teaspoon thyme
½	red bell pepper, cubed
½	onion, chopped and peeled blade #3
4	large baking potatoes, about ¼ pound (345 g) each, cut 1-inch cubes
1	tablespoon fresh parsley, chopped

In the 4-quart Stockpot (4 L), melt butter in olive oil over medium heat. Add all ingredients and toss to coat. Cover, close the vent, reduce the heat to medium-low heat, form the vapor seal, and cook the waterless way about 35-40 minutes.

To serve, spoon to serving bowl toss gently, and top with chopped parsley.

NUTRITIONAL BREAKDOWN PER SERVING: Calories 150; Fat Grams 3; Carbohydrate Grams 28; Protein Grams 3; Cholesterol mg 4; Sodium mg 24.

THE POINT SYSTEM: Calorie Points 2; Protein Points 0; Fat Grams 3; Sodium Points 1; Fiber Points 1; Carbohydrate Points 2; Cholesterol Points 0.

Vegetable Curry

Serves: 8
Preparation Time: 40 minutes
Equipment: small stainless mixing bowl, French chef knife, cutting board,
Kitchen Machine food cutter, 6-quart stockpot

3	tablespoons curry spice mix, see recipe page 205
3	tablespoons vinegar
¼	cup (60 ml) peanut oil
2	onions, chopped and peeled blade #3
2	cloves garlic, minced
4	¾ pound (345 g) baking potatoes cut into 2-inch cubes
I	pound mushrooms, quartered
½	teaspoon sea salt or kosher salt
I	16 ounce (460 g) can diced tomatoes
	or I¼-pounds plum tomatoes, peeled, seeded and diced
I	cup (240 ml) unsweetened coconut milk
½	teaspoon Garam Masala, see recipe page 205
I	8 ounce (230 g) package frozen peas

In a small mixing bowl, combine the curry spice mix with vinegar, mix to form into a paste, set aside.

In the 6-quart stockpot, heat peanut oil over medium heat. Add onions and garlic, sauté until golden brown. Add curry spice/vinegar spice mixture and fry for about 3-minutes stirring constantly. Add potatoes and mushrooms, salt, and mix well. Cover, close the vent, and reduce the heat to low, about 20 minutes.

Add tomatoes, cover and simmer an additional 5 minutes. Add coconut milk, Garam Masala, and peas. Stir, cover, and simmer uncovered until heated through.

Serve with Raita and Chicken Satay.

NUTRITIONAL BREAKDOWN PER SERVING: Calories 264; Fat Grams 15; Carbohydrate Grams 30; Protein Grams 6; Cholesterol mg 0; Sodium mg 268 (161 with fresh tomatoes).

THE POINT SYSTEM: Calorie Points 3½; Protein Points 1; Fat Grams 15; Sodium Points 12 (8 with fresh tomatoes); Fiber Points 2; Carbohydrate Points 2; Cholesterol Points 0.

Vegetarian Spring Rolls

Serves: 8
Preparation Time: 40 minutes
Equipment: French chef knife, cutting board, Kitchen Machine food cutter,
medium mixing Bowl, small mixing bowl, 13-inch chef pan or 6-quart stockpot with
steamer rack, and 4½-quart Dutch oven cover

2	ounces (60 g) bean threads (soaked in warm water about 10 minutes)
1	cup carrots, grated blade #1
1	red onion, chopped and peeled blade #3
1	small head green cabbage, chopped fine blade #2
1	red pepper, chopped
1½	tablespoons garlic, minced
1	tablespoon soy sauce
1	teaspoon fresh ginger, grated blade #1
2	eggs, beaten
1	tablespoon cornstarch
1	package spring roll wrappers

Using the food cutter, cut carrots, red onion, and green cabbage into medium mixing bowl, add chopped red pepper, garlic, soy sauce, ginger and beaten eggs. Mix well.

In the small mixing bowl, combine ½ cup (120 ml) water and 1 tablespoon cornstarch, mix well, (will be used to seal edges of spring rolls).

Place about 2 tablespoons of vegetables mixture one-third the way up the spring roll wrapper, fold corners over filling, roll to form a lightly packed log shaped roll. Seal edges with cornstarch and water mixture. If wrappers dry out, lightly dampen with a sprinkle of water prior to filling.

TO FRY: In the 13-inch (33 cm) chef pan, bring 2-inches of oil to temperature over medium heat. Fry 2 to 3 stuffed rolls at a time until they are firm and golden brown.

TO STEAM: In the 6-quart stockpot, bring 2 to 3-inches of water to a boil. Spray steamer rack with cooking spray, place spring rolls on steamer rack, cover with 4½-quart Dutch oven cover and steam to heat through. To keep hot leave Dutch oven cover on, turn off heat, and Spring Rolls will remain warm for 1 hour.

Serve with Soy Dipping Sauce, see recipe page 159

NUTRITIONAL BREAKDOWN PER SERVING: Calories 69; Fat Grams 0; Carbohydrate Grams 14; Protein Grams 4; Cholesterol mg 0; Sodium mg 180.

THE POINT SYSTEM: Calorie Points 1; Protein Points ½; Fat Grams 0; Sodium Points 8; Fiber Points 2; Carbohydrate Points 1; Cholesterol Points 0.

Soy Dipping Sauce

Yields: 2 cups
Preparation Time: 10 minutes
Equipment: small stainless mixing bowl, French chef knife, cutting board

½	cup (120 ml) water
½	cup (120 ml) white distiller vinegar or rice vinegar
½	cup (120 ml) soy sauce
½	cup raw sugar or sugar substitute
1	teaspoon chili paste
2	teaspoons garlic, minced fine

In the mixing bowl, combine all ingredients.

Nutritional breakdown includes sugar.

NUTRITIONAL BREAKDOWN PER SERVING: Calories 71; Fat Grams 0; Carbohydrate Grams 17; Protein Grams 2; Cholesterol mg 0; Sodium mg 538.

THE POINT SYSTEM: Calorie Points 1; Protein Points 1; Fat Grams 0; Sodium Points 23; Fiber Points 0; Carbohydrate Points 1; Cholesterol Points 0.

Stuffed Artichokes

Serves: 4
Preparation Time: 45 minutes
Equipment: French chef knife, cutting board, Kitchen Machine food cutter, medium stainless mixing bowl, 6-quart stockpot, steamer rack, Dutch oven cover

4	artichokes
I	fresh lemon, juice thereof
I¼	cups Italian bread crumbs
I	clove garlic, minced
¼	cup parsley, chopped
¼	cup Parmesan cheese, grated blade #1
¼	teaspoon dried basil, or ½ teaspoon fresh basil, chopped
2	tablespoons olive oil
2	tablespoons dry white wine

Wash and trim stems and remove loose outer leaves from artichokes. Cut off ½-inch (1.5 cm) from top, and snip off leaf tips with kitchen shears. Brush edges with lemon juice.

In the mixing bowl, combine remaining ingredients. Starting at the bottom of the artichoke and working up, place a small amount stuffing in between each artichoke leaf.

In the 6-quart stockpot with the steamer rack on top, bring 2 cups of water to a boil. Place artichokes on steamer rack, cover with the Dutch oven cover, reduce the heat to medium-low, and steam artichokes about 30 minutes or until leaf pulls off easily.

NUTRITIONAL BREAKDOWN PER SERVING: Calories 357; Fat Grams 11; Carbohydrate Grams 52; Protein Grams 20; Cholesterol mg 5; Sodium mg 777.

THE POINT SYSTEM: Calorie Points 5; Protein Points 2½; Fat Grams 11; Sodium Points 34; Fiber Points 9; Carbohydrate Points 3½; Cholesterol Points ½.

Skillet Cabbage

Serves: 8
Preparation Time: 30 minutes
Equipment: French chef knife, cutting board, Kitchen Machine food cutter, large skillet

2	slices bacon or Canadian bacon, chopped (optional)
4	cups red cabbage, shredded blade #5
1	green pepper cut in strips
2	cups celery diced
2	medium onions, quartered, julienned and peeled blade #2
2	tomatoes cut in half with each half cut in quarters
2	teaspoons raw sugar

In the large skillet brown bacon over medium heat, remove bacon to paper towels. Reduce heat to medium-low; add cabbage, green pepper, celery and onion. Cover, close the vent, and cook 15 minutes. Stir in tomatoes and sugar, cover and cook an additional 10-15 minutes.

NUTRITIONAL BREAKDOWN PER SERVING: Calories 64; Fat Grams 1; Carbohydrate Grams 13; Protein Grams 2; Cholesterol mg 1; Sodium mg 60.

THE POINT SYSTEM: Calorie Points 1; Protein Points 0; Fat Grams 1; Sodium Points 3; Fiber Points 2; Carbohydrate Points 1; Cholesterol Points 0.

Grains, Pastas,

Beans & Breads...

Italian Focaccia

Serves: 8
Preparation Time: 1 hour 50 minutes
(1 hour 30 minutes rising time)
Equipment: large stainless mixing bowl, 13-inch chef pan

Focaccia is as flavorful a simple country bread can get. Olive oil and rosemary give this yeast-raised flatbread its glorious Italian flavor.

1	package active dried yeast
1	cup (240 ml) warm water
2½	tablespoons fresh rosemary, sniped
3	tablespoons olive oil
2	teaspoons salt
2½-3	cups all purpose flour
	Coarsely ground black pepper (optional)

In the mixing bowl, dissolve yeast in warm water. Stir in rosemary, olive oil, salt and enough flour to make dough easy to handle. Turn dough onto lightly floured surface; knead until smooth and elastic, 5-10 minutes. Place in greased bowl; turn greased side up, cover and let rise in a warm place until in doubles in size, about 1 hour. (Dough is ready when indentation remains when untouched.)

Punch down dough. Press into oiled 13-inch (33 cm) chef pan. On top of dough, make depressions with fingers, about 2" (5 cm) apart. Brush with oil and sprinkle with pepper. Let rise uncovered, about 30 minutes. Cover, close the vent, and bake on medium heat, about 15 minutes. Reduce heat to low and continue to cook covered with the vent closed 10 more minutes. Bake until golden brown, check when done by gently lifting the bottom with a spatula. Brush with additional oil and serve warm.

NOTE: for darker crust on the top, after the first 15 minutes of cooking time on top of the stove, the chef pan can be placed in the oven without the cover and finished cooking at 375°F (190°C) for 10 minutes.

To serve, top with coarsely ground fresh black pepper.

NUTRITIONAL BREAKDOWN PER SERVING: Calories 288; Fat Grams 6; Carbohydrate Grams 46; Protein Grams 13; Cholesterol mg 0; Sodium mg 547.

THE POINT SYSTEM: Calorie Points 4; Protein Points 0; Fat Grams 6; Sodium Points 24; Fiber Points 3; Carbohydrate Points 3; Cholesterol Points 0.

Dutch Babies

Serves: 6
Preparation Time: 35 minutes
Equipment: 13-inch chef pan, large stainless mixing bowl

⅓	cup unsalted butter
4	whole eggs
I	cup (240 ml) skim milk
I	cup flour
	Ground nutmeg

Melt butter in 13-inch chef pan in preheated 400°F (210°C) oven. While butter melts, mix batter.

In the large mixing bowl, whisk eggs until blended and foamy, blend in milk and flour. Remove pan from oven and pour in batter. Return pan to oven and bake until puffy and well browned (20-25 minutes).

Dust pancake with ground nutmeg and serve hot with toppings listed below.

POWDERED SUGAR CLASSIC
Have a shaker or bowl of powdered sugar and thick wedges of lemon ready. Sprinkle powdered sugar on hot pancake, squeeze on fresh lemon juice and serve.

FRUIT
Sliced strawberries and peaches sweetened to taste or any fruit in season, cut and sweetened.

SYRUP
Top with warm or cold honey, maple syrup, or any favorite fruit syrup or sauce.

NUTRITIONAL BREAKDOWN PER SERVING: Calories 192; Fat Grams 10; Carbohydrate Grams 18; Protein Grams 6; Cholesterol mg 28; Sodium mg 162.

THE POINT SYSTEM: Calorie Points 2½; Protein Points I; Fat Grams 10; Sodium Points 7; Fiber Points 0; Carbohydrate Points I; Cholesterol Points 3.

Cornbread

On top of the stove
Serves: 16
Preparation Time: 50 minutes
Equipment: large stainless mixing bowl, large skillet

2	whole eggs
4	cups white self-rising cornmeal
3	cups (720 ml) 1% milk
4	tablespoons raw sugar
2	tablespoons unsalted butter or margarine

In the mixing bowl, whisk eggs until frothy, add flour, milk, sugar, and mix well. Melt butter in the large skillet over medium heat, coat the bottom and sides. Pour the batter in the pan, reduce to low heat, cover, close the vent, and bake for about 35-45 minutes. Test for doneness with toothpick.

NOTE: A tip when baking on top of the stove. When removing the lid, invert immediately and move away from over the top of what's baking. The moisture condenses on the lid and will drip when vapor seal is broken.

NUTRITIONAL BREAKDOWN PER SERVING: Calories 162; Fat Grams 2; Carbohydrate Grams 31; Protein Grams 5; Cholesterol mg 2; Sodium mg 511.

THE POINT SYSTEM: Calorie Points 2; Protein Points 1; Fat Grams 2; Sodium Points 22; Fiber Points 1; Carbohydrate Points 2; Cholesterol Points 0.

Griddle Oat Scones

Serves: 8
Preparation Time: 20 minutes
Equipment: large stainless mixing bowl, 13-inch chef pan

I	cup quick rolled oats
I	cup all-purpose flour
½	teaspoon salt
2	teaspoons baking powder
I	teaspoon baking soda
¼	cup cold unsalted butter
⅔	cup (160 ml) buttermilk

In the large mixing bowl, combine oats, flour, salt, baking powder and baking soda. Using a pastry blender or fork, cut the butter in with the flour mixture until it looks like coarse crumbs. Stir in the buttermilk until the dough holds together.

On a floured surface knead the dough, and then form into a ball. Flatten it to a circle, about ½-inch (1.5 cm) thick. With a knife, cut dough into 8 pie-shaped wedges.

Rub a small amount of flour on a cold, 13-inch chef pan. Heat the pan on medium-low heat for 5 minutes. Place scone wedges in the pan and cook 6-8 minutes on each side. Turn only once.

To serve, top hot with fruit preserves or Frozen Strawberry Jam, recipe page 146.

NUTRITIONAL BREAKDOWN PER SERVING: Calories 156; Fat Grams 7; Carbohydrate Grams 20; Protein Grams 4; Cholesterol mg 16; Sodium mg 444.

THE POINT SYSTEM: Calorie Points 2; Protein Points ½; Fat Grams 7; Sodium Points 19; Fiber Points 1; Carbohydrate Points 1½; Cholesterol Points 2.

Nan Bread

Baked Leavened Bread from India
Serves: 4
Preparation Time: 45 minutes
Equipment: large stainless mixing bowl, 1-quart saucepan, 10-inch chef pan

1	cup whole meal wheat flour
1	teaspoon raw sugar
½	teaspoon baking powder
½	teaspoon salt
3	tablespoons milk
¼	cup plain yogurt
1	ounce (30 g) yeast dissolved in a little bit of milk
2	tablespoons unsalted butter, melted or 1 egg yoke
1	tablespoon poppy seeds

Sift flour, sugar, baking powder and salt into large mixing bowl.

In the 1-quart saucepan, warm milk and yogurt on low heat, add yeast, butter and egg. Whisk to combine thoroughly.

Make a depression in the center of flour and pour milk mixture a little at a time until all is absorbed. On floured surface knead well for about 15 minutes until smooth and springy, adding a little more flour if the dough is sticky. Cover and leave to rise until double in bulk size (approximately 2 hours, unless weather is hot, in which case dough might rise in half the time).

Divide into 8 equal portions, with well flour hands roll into balls. Cover and set aside, about 15 minutes. Flatten each ball into a thick pancake. With the help of a little flour, toss from one palm to the other.

To bake, brush tops with melted butter or beaten egg yolk, sprinkle with poppy seeds. Cook in preheated 10-inch chef pan or skillet on medium-heat; when first side is browned, flip and brown the other side.

Serve with Hummus, recipe page 80.

NUTRITIONAL BREAKDOWN PER SERVING: Calories 343; Fat Grams 10; Carbohydrate Grams 51; Protein Grams 16; Cholesterol mg 69; Sodium mg 435.

THE POINT SYSTEM: Calorie Points 4½; Protein Points 2; Fat Grams 10; Sodium Points 19; Fiber Points 3; Carbohydrate Points 3½; Cholesterol Points 7.

Basmati Pea Pilaf

Matar Polao
Serves: 6
Preparation Time: 1 hour 15 minutes
Equipment: French chef knife, cutting board, 6-quart stockpot, 1-quart saucepan

1	cup basmati rice
2	cups (480 ml) water
½	teaspoon sea salt or kosher salt
2	tablespoons olive oil
3	tablespoons unsalted butter
1	small onion, sliced
2	teaspoons Garam Masala, see spice recipe page 204
2	cups (480 ml) water
½	cup golden raisins
½	cup frozen peas
¼	cup blanched almonds, see recipe page 205
2	tablespoons chopped green onions

Rinse basmati rice then soak for 1 hour in 2 cups of water with salt added. Drain rice (which is now very brittle) be careful not to break it.

While rice is soaking, heat oil and butter in 6-quart (6L) stockpot over medium heat. Add onions and sauté until light golden brown. Add raisins and sauté 5 minutes. Remove raisins and a few onions for garnish.

In a 1-quart saucepan, bring 2 cups of water to a boil and stir in Garam Masala (blend of spices). After removing raisins from onion, butter mixture, add boiling spice mixture to 6-quart stockpot, add rice, but do not stir. Bring to a boil, 7-10 minutes, reduce to low, sprinkle in peas, cover, close the vent, and cook an additional 5-10 minutes.

To serve, spoon rice mixture onto large platter, garnish with reserved onions and raisins, top with blanched almonds and green onions.

NUTRITIONAL BREAKDOWN PER SERVING: Calories 350; Fat Grams 18; Carbohydrate Grams 42; Protein Grams 9; Cholesterol mg 10; Sodium mg 233.

THE POINT SYSTEM: Calorie Points 4½; Protein Points 1; Fat Grams 18; Sodium Points 10; Fiber Points 2; Carbohydrate Points 3; Cholesterol Points 1.

Hom Bow

Yields: 10 buns
Preparation Time: 15 minutes
(1 hour rising time)
Cooking Time: 15 to 25 minutes
Equipment: French chef knife, cutting board, Kitchen Machine food cutter,
2-quart saucepan, large stainless mixing bowl with cover, small stainless mixing bowl,
large skillet, steamer rack, 4½-quart Dutch oven cover.

1¼	cups (300 ml) skim milk
1	tablespoon active dry yeast
1	tablespoon raw sugar
1	tablespoon vegetable oil
½	teaspoon salt
3½	cups (approximately) all purpose flour

FILLING

2	tablespoons onion, diced, blade #2
1	clove garlic, minced
1	tablespoon peanut oil
½	pound (230 g) lean ground pork
⅓	cup (80 ml) water
2	tablespoons soy sauce
2	teaspoons cornstarch
2	teaspoons raw sugar
½	teaspoon fresh grated ginger, blade #1

In the 2-quart saucepan (2 L) heat milk until warm, stir in yeast, sugar, oil, and salt, mix well. Add ½ the flour and blend together thoroughly, stir in enough remaining flour to make dough soft for kneading. Knead lightly on floured surface. Return to lightly greased large mixing bowl, turning ounce to grease surface. Cover and let rise in a warm place until double in size (approximately 45-60 minutes).

In small mixing bowl, stir together water and soy sauce into cornstarch, add sugar and ginger, mix well and set aside.

In the 2-quart Saucepan (2 L), over medium heat, sauté onion and garlic in peanut oil until tender (do not brown). Add the ground pork, sauté until cooked through. Add water/soy sauce mixture, stir until thickened, and remove from heat. Cover and cool in refrigerator until ready to use.

When rising period has finished, punch the dough down, turn onto lightly floured surface and shape into 10 balls. Cover and let rest 5 minutes.

On a lightly floured surface, flatten each ball of dough to about a 3½-inch (9cm) circle. Place a rounded spoonful of pork mixture in center of each circle of dough. Bring edges of dough up around filling, stretching until edges meet, and pinch to seal.

TO STEAM
Place 1 cup (240 ml) water in large skillet. With a (greased) 10-inch steamer rack placed in the skillet bring water to a boil and place the buns on the rack, cover with 4.5-quart Dutch oven cover and steam over medium heat about 15 minutes.

TO BAKE
Place buns in greased 13-inch chef pan or double griddle. Bake in 375°F (190°C) oven for 25 minutes, or until golden brown.

NUTRITIONAL BREAKDOWN PER SERVING: Calories 265; Fat Grams 8; Carbohydrate Grams 39; Protein Grams 10; Cholesterol mg 14; Sodium mg 484.

THE POINT SYSTEM: Calorie Points 3½; Protein Points 1; Fat Grams 8; Sodium Points 0; Fiber Points 0; Carbohydrate Points 2½; Cholesterol Points 1.

Spicy Wehani Rice with Cashews

Serves: 6
Preparation Time: 50 minutes
Equipment: French chef knife, cutting board, Kitchen Machine food cutter, 3-quart saucepan

¼	cup chicken broth or homemade chicken stock
2	teaspoons cumin seed
¼	teaspoon ground cloves
I	bay leaf
¼	teaspoon hot pepper flakes
I	medium onion, halved, chopped and peeled blade #3
2	cloves garlic, minced
I	cup Wehani Rice, uncooked
2¼	cups (540 ml) hot water
½	teaspoon salt
¼	cup roasted cashews, chopped

In the 3-quart (3 L) saucepan, heat the chicken stock over medium heat, add the cumin seed, cloves and bay leaf, stir until fragrant about 15-20 seconds. Add the red pepper, onion and garlic, sauté until softened. Stir in the rice and coat, cook about 2 minutes. Add water and salt, stir, cover, close the vent, and reduce heat to low. Do not remove the cover lid for about 40 minutes. Remove from heat and let stand covered another 15 minutes. Remove bay leaf.

To serve, stir in cashews just before serving.

NUTRITIONAL BREAKDOWN PER SERVING: Calories 130; Fat Grams 5; Carbohydrate Grams 19; Protein Grams 4; Cholesterol mg 0; Sodium mg 311.

THE POINT SYSTEM: Calorie Points 1½; Protein Points 0; Fat Grams 5; Sodium Points 14; Fiber Points I; Carbohydrate Points I; Cholesterol Points 0.

Couscous with Chicken Thighs

Serves: 4

Preparation Time: 50 minutes

Equipment: French chef knife, cutting board, Kitchen Machine food cutter, large skillet

2	tablespoons olive oil
I	teaspoon ground cinnamon
I	teaspoon cumin
I	teaspoon paprika
4	chicken thighs, skinned
I	onion, sliced thin
I	cup parsnips, sliced blade #4
¼	cup carrots, sliced blade #4
½	cup celery, sliced blade #4
I0	dried apricots halves
I	I5 ounce (430 g) can diced tomatoes
	or I¼ pounds fresh plum tomatoes, peeled, seeded and diced
3	cups (720 ml) water
I¼	cups couscous
2	tablespoons cilantro, chopped

In the large skillet, preheat olive oil over medium heat. Add cinnamon, cumin, and paprika, stir until fragrant. Add chicken thighs, turn heat to low, cover, open the vent, sauté 5-7 minutes. Turn chicken, add onion, parsnips, carrots, celery and apricots, cover and cook about 5 minutes. Add the tomatoes and water, cover and simmer 30 minutes. Remove from heat, place chicken on platter and keep warm. Add couscous to skillet, cover and let stand about 5 minutes.

To serve, spoon couscous onto center of platter, surround with chicken thighs, and topped with chopped cilantro.

NUTRITIONAL BREAKDOWN PER SERVING: Calories 4I5; Fat Grams I4; Carbohydrate Grams 56; Protein Grams 20; Cholesterol mg 49; Sodium mg 295 (I77 with fresh tomatoes).

THE POINT SYSTEM: Calorie Points 5½; Protein Points 3; Fat Grams I4; Sodium Points I3 (8 if fresh tomatoes); Fiber Points 5; Carbohydrate Points 4; Cholesterol Points 5.

Chinese "Not Fried" Rice

Serves: 6
Preparation Time: 35 minutes
Equipment: French chef knife, cutting board, Kitchen Machine food cutter, 2-quart saucepan

I	small onion, halved, chopped and peeled blade #3
2	cups (480 ml) chicken broth, or homemade chicken stock
I	tablespoon, dry Sherry, or dry white wine
I	tablespoon soy sauce
I	teaspoon sesame seed oil
I	cup uncooked long grain or brown rice
½	cup green onions, diagonally sliced
I	tablespoon pine nuts, toasted

In the 2-quart (2 L) saucepan over medium heat, dry sauté onion, covered until tender, about 2-3 minutes. Add chicken stock, sherry, soy sauce, sesame seed oil and bring to a boil over medium-high heat. Stir in rice, cover, close the vent, reduce heat to low, cook 25 minutes or until rice is tender and liquid is absorbed. Remove from heat and stir in green onions and pine nuts.

NUTRITIONAL BREAKDOWN PER SERVING: Calories 86; Fat Grams 2; Carbohydrate Grams 11; Protein Grams 3; Cholesterol mg 0; Sodium mg 432 (259 with homemade chicken stock).

THE POINT SYSTEM: Calorie Points 1; Protein Points 0; Fat Grams 2; Sodium Points 19 (12 with homemade chicken stock); Fiber Points 0; Carbohydrate Points 2; Cholesterol Points ½.

Pasta Puttánesca

Serves: 6

Preparation Time: 50 minutes

Equipment: French chef knife, cutting board, Kitchen Machine food cutter, 2-quart saucepan, 6½-quart 'Tall' stockpot, 6-quart pasta/steamer basket

3	tablespoons olive oil
½	small onion, chopped and peeled blade #5
2	cloves garlic, minced
1½	cups (360 ml) can Italian plum tomatoes
	or fresh plum tomatoes, peeled, seeded and chopped
4	quarts (4 L) water
½	teaspoon sea salt or kosher salt
1	pound (460 g) rigatoni, penne or fusilli pasta, cooked
1	tablespoon capers
½	cup black olives, chopped
3	tablespoon fresh basil, chopped
1	teaspoon dried red pepper flakes
½	cup Romano cheese, grated blade #1
1	tablespoon fresh basil, chopped

In the 2-quart (2 L) saucepan, preheat oil over medium heat; add onion and garlic, and sauté until transparent. Reduce heat to low, add tomatoes, cover, open vent, and simmer 25 minutes.

While the sauce in simmering; in the 6½-quart stockpot with 6-quart pasta/steamer basket inserted, bring 4-quarts of water to a boil, and add salt and pasta. Cook until al dente (firm to the bite). Remove pasta/steamer insert to drain. Pour pasta into serving bowl.

Add capers, olives, basil and red pepper flakes, to sauce, mix well, and simmer an additional 5 minutes.

To serve, spoon sauce over pasta, toss gently, top with grated Romano cheese and chopped basil.

NUTRITIONAL BREAKDOWN PER SERVING: Calories 371; Fat Grams 16; Carbohydrate Grams 48; Protein Grams 13; Cholesterol mg 101; Sodium mg 326 (196 with fresh plum tomatoes).

THE POINT SYSTEM: Calorie Points 5; Protein Points 2; Fat Grams 16; Sodium Points 14 (9 with fresh plum tomatoes); Fiber Points 1; Carbohydrate Points 3; Cholesterol Points 10.

Pasta Carbonaro

Serves: 10
Preparation Time: 30 minutes
Equipment: French chef knife, cutting board, Kitchen Machine food cutter, 6½-quart stockpot,
6-quart pasta/steamer basket

½	teaspoon sea salt or kosher salt
I	pound (460 g) penne pasta
½	pound (230 g) pancetta cut in ½-inch (1.5 cm) slices*
½	cup Romano cheese, grated blade #I
¼	cup Parmesan cheese, grated blade #I
4	whole eggs, beaten
I	tablespoon fresh parsley, chopped

In the 6½-quart stockpot, with 6-quart pasta/steamer basket inserted, bring 4 quarts of water to a boil. Add salt and pasta, cook until al dente (firm to the bite). Remove pasta/steamer basket to drain.

In the 6½-quart stockpot, sauté pancetta over medium heat until it clarifies, add cooked pasta, stir well, and remove from heat. Slowly add cheeses, stirring well. Add eggs, stirring quickly to keep from curdling.

To serve, garnish with parsley.

NOTE*: if pancetta (Italian bacon) is not available, substitute with sliced bacon, sautéed until almost crisp.

NUTRITIONAL BREAKDOWN PER SERVING: Calories 294; Fat Grams 9; Carbohydrate Grams 35; Protein Grams 18; Cholesterol mg 28; Sodium mg 332.

THE POINT SYSTEM: Calorie Points 4; Protein Points 2; Fat Grams 8; Sodium Points 14; Fiber Points I; Carbohydrate Points 2½; Cholesterol Points 3.

Pasta Shrimp Salad

Serves: 4
Preparation Time: 30 minutes
Equipment: French chef knife, cutting board, Kitchen Machine food cutter

3	celery ribs, chopped
3	sweet pickles, chopped
3	hard cooked eggs, chopped, see recipe for waterless hard cooked eggs page 31
2	green onions, chopped
1½	cups cooked shrimp, peeled and deveined
3	cups cooked pasta shells or tortellini
3	cups fresh pineapple tidbits and juice
½	cup fat free mayonnaise
½	head lettuce, shredded
1	green onion, chopped

In a large salad bowl, combine all ingredients except lettuce. Place lettuce in pineapple cavity, spoon in salad mixture.

To serve, top with chopped green onions.

NUTRITIONAL BREAKDOWN PER SERVING: Calories 299; Fat Grams 5; Carbohydrate Grams 50; Protein Grams 13; Cholesterol mg 187; Sodium mg 581.

THE POINT SYSTEM: Calorie Points 4; Protein Points 2; Fat Grams 5; Sodium Points 25; Fiber Points 1; Carbohydrate Points 3½; Cholesterol Points 19.

Pasta Primavera

Serves: 8
Yields: 2 quarts (2 L)
Preparation Time: 30 minutes
Equipment: French chef knife, cutting board, Kitchen Machine food cutter,
medium skillet, 6.5-quart "Tall" stockpot, 6-quart steamer/pasta insert,
1-quart saucepan, small stainless Mixing Bowl

¼	pound (115 g) fresh mushrooms, sliced blade #4 (to slice, lay sideways in hopper)
1	clove garlic, minced fine or pureed to a paste with side of knife blade
½	cup broccoli florets
½	cup fresh snow pea pods
½	cup yellow squash, sliced blade #4 or waffle sliced blade #5
½	cup zucchini, sliced blade #4 or waffle sliced blade #5
1	tablespoon fresh chives, chopped
8	ounces (230 g) fresh linguini, uncooked
¼	cup (60 ml) hot water
2	tablespoons Chablis or another dry white wine
¼	teaspoon chicken bouillon
¼	cup (180 ml) skim milk
1	tablespoons all purpose flour
¼	cup Parmesan cheese, plus 1 tablespoon, grated blade #1
1	tablespoon fresh parsley, chopped
1½	tablespoons fresh basil, chopped

In the medium skillet, sweat down mushrooms over medium heat, about 4-5 minutes, stir occasionally. Add garlic, snow peas, yellow squash, zucchini, chives, cover, close the vent, reduce heat to low, form the vapor seal and cook waterless 15-20 minutes.

In the 6.5-quart stockpot with 6-quart pasta/steamer inserted, cook linguini according to package directions. Drain and set aside.

In the 1-quart (1 L) saucepan, combine water, wine and bouillon; bring to a simmer over medium-high heat. In the small mixing bowl, combine milk and flour, mix well. Gradually add to water and wine mixture, stirring constantly until sauce bubbles and thickens.

To serve, place linguini in large serving bowl, pour sauce over pasta and toss gently. Add Parmesan cheese, parsley and basil, toss. Top with vegetable mixture, and remaining Parmesan cheese.

NUTRITIONAL BREAKDOWN PER SERVING: Calories 80; Fat Grams 1; Carbohydrate Grams 12; Protein Grams 5; Cholesterol mg 12; Sodium mg 75.

THE POINT SYSTEM: Calorie Points 1; Protein Points ½; Fat Grams 1; Sodium Points 3; Fiber Points 0; Carbohydrate Points 1; Cholesterol Points 1.

Reduced Calorie Fettuccini

Serves: 12 – 1 cup servings
Preparation Time: 20 minutes
Equipment: French chef knife, cutting board, Kitchen Machine food cutter, 6-quart pasta/
steamer unit, 6.5-quart 'Tall' stockpot

1	package, about 12 ounces (460 g) fettuccini pasta
½	cup plain yogurt or low-fat yogurt
½	cup Parmesan cheese, grated blade #1
1	tablespoon fresh ground black pepper
2	tablespoons fresh parsley, chopped

Using the 6-quart pasta/steamer unit inserted into the 6.5-quart Stockpot, fill with water and bring to a boil over medium high heat. Add fettuccini and salt (optional), and cook until al dente (firm to the bite). Remove Pasta insert and drain.

To serve, place hot pasta in a large serving bowl. Add yogurt, Parmesan cheese, black pepper, toss, and top with chopped parsley.

NUTRITIONAL BREAKDOWN PER SERVING: Calories 75; Fat Grams 2; Carbohydrate Grams 11; Protein Grams 4; Cholesterol mg 16; Sodium mg 265.

THE POINT SYSTEM: Calorie Points 1; Protein Points ½; Fat Grams 2; Sodium Points 12; Fiber Points 0; Carbohydrate Points ½; Cholesterol Points 1½.

Garlic Bread

Serves: 12
Preparation Time: 10 minutes
Equipment: French chef knife, cutting board, double griddle, 8-inch chef pan

4	cloves garlic, minced fine
¼	cup diet margarine or unsalted butter
I	loaf Italian, French or Cuban bread, sliced

Preheat double griddle over medium heat. In the 8-inch chef pan sauté garlic in margarine or butter over medium heat 2-3 minutes and remove from heat. Using a pastry brush, lightly brush one side of bread with butter/garlic mixture and place on double griddle, buttered side down. Cook each piece about 2 minutes until golden brown, turn and lightly toast unbuttered side.

Serve alone with pasta, or top with Salsa (see recipe page 102) for an excellent Bruschetta.

NUTRITIONAL BREAKDOWN PER SERVING: Calories 86; Fat Grams 3; Carbohydrate Grams 13; Protein Grams 2; Cholesterol mg 0; Sodium mg 196.

THE POINT SYSTEM: Calorie Points 1; Protein Points 0; Fat Grams 3; Sodium Points 9; Fiber Points 0; Carbohydrate Points 1; Cholesterol Points 0.

Soda Bread

Yields: 2 dozen
Preparation Time: 1 hour 10 minutes
Equipment: large stainless mixing bowl, large skillet, 10-inch chef pan

4	cups flour
1	teaspoon baking soda
1	teaspoon salt
1	tablespoon unsalted butter
½	cup (120 ml) buttermilk
½	cup raisins (optional)

Sift flour, baking soda and salt into large mixing bowl. Cut in butter with a fork or pastry cutter. Add buttermilk and stir. Knead dough for several minutes on a floured surface. Form into 2-inch balls; flatten slightly. Using a floured knife, cut slits in tops of dough balls. Place in ungreased large skillet and cover with inverted 10-inch chef skillet to form a high dome cover, bake over low heat for 45 minutes or until done. Serve with honey.

NUTRITIONAL BREAKDOWN PER SERVING: Calories 246; Fat Grams 2; Carbohydrate Grams 48; Protein Grams 7; Cholesterol mg 4; Sodium mg 456.

THE POINT SYSTEM: Calorie Points 3½; Protein Points 1; Fat Grams 2; Sodium Points 19; Fiber Points 1; Carbohydrate Points 3; Cholesterol Points 0.

Desserts. . .

Chocolate Glazed Poached Pears

Serves: 6
Preparation Time: 45 minutes
Equipment: 6-quart stockpot, stainless cookie sheet, 11-inch wok/saucier

6	firm but ripe pears
3	tablespoons (45 ml) water
3	ounces (90 g) German sweet chocolate, chopped
3	ounces (90 g) semisweet chocolate, chopped
¼	cup unsalted butter
18	mint leaves for garnish

PEARS

If skin is thick, using a vegetable peeler, peel pears and leave stems intact. If not thick, do not peel. If necessary, cut a small slice off each pear's bottom so it will stand upright.

Place pears in the 6-quart (6 L) stockpot or large skillet, add 3 tablespoons water, cover and close the vent. Place over low heat for 30 minutes. Remove pears with a slotted spoon and place on cookie sheet to cool. Pears may be refrigerated several hours (or overnight) if desired.

GLAZE

A few hours before serving, melt both varieties of chocolate and butter in 11-inch wok/saucier over medium-low heat, whisk until ingredients are combined and heated through. When smooth, remove from heat.

Blot all pears dry with paper towels and line cookie sheet with wax paper. Holding each pear carefully by the stem, dip into the chocolate glazing mixture, tilting pear and spooning glaze to cover completely. Place on cooking sheet and refrigerate for several hours.

To serve, remove pears to serving plate with spatula, and garnish with mint leaves.

Alternative, leaving stems intact, wash strawberries, blot dry with paper towel, dip in chocolate sauce, place on a wax paper lined cookie sheet and refrigerate for 1-2 hours before serving.

NUTRITIONAL BREAKDOWN PER SERVING: Calories 308; Fat Grams 18; Carbohydrate Grams 42; Protein Grams 2; Cholesterol mg 10; Sodium mg 71.

THE POINT SYSTEM: Calorie Points 4; Protein Points 0; Fat Grams 18; Sodium Points 3; Fiber Points 3; Carbohydrate Points 34; Cholesterol Points 1.

Fruit and Ginger Pears

Serves: 6
Preparation Time: 50 minutes
Equipment: 6-quart stockpot, small stainless mixing bowl

6	medium pears
1	8 ¾ ounce (250 g) can fruit cocktail, drained, reserving syrup to measuring cup
¼	cup (60 ml) fresh squeezed orange juice
2	teaspoon crystallized ginger, chopped or fresh ginger, grated blade #1
1	tablespoon cornstarch
1	tablespoon water
3	tablespoons dry sherry

Add enough water to syrup from fruit cocktail to make 2/3 cup (160 ml) of liquid. In the 6-quart (6 L) stockpot or large skillet, combine reserved syrup/water mixture, orange juice, and ginger. Place pears upright in liquid and bring to simmer over medium to medium-high heat. Reduce heat to low, cover, close the vent, and cook 40 minutes. Remove pears to individual serving bowls.

In the small mixing bowl, combine cornstarch and water, mix well. Stir cornstarch/water mixture into hot syrup, stirring until mixture thickens. Remove from heat and stir in sherry and fruit cocktail.

To serve, spoon fruit cocktail sauce over pears, can be served warm or cold.

NUTRITIONAL BREAKDOWN PER SERVING: Calories 173; Fat Grams 1; Carbohydrate Grams 41; Protein Grams 1; Cholesterol mg 0; Sodium mg 8.

THE POINT SYSTEM: Calorie Points 2½; Protein Points 0; Fat Grams 1; Sodium Points 0; Fiber Points 2; Carbohydrate Points 2½; Cholesterol Points 0.

Marbled Brownies

Yields: 2 dozen
Preparation Time: 30 minutes
Equipment: 2 large stainless mixing bowls, electric mixer, large skillet or 13-inch (33 cm) chef pan

¼	cup + 2 tablespoons diet margarine or unsalted butter, softened
½	cup cream cheese, softened
½	cup raw sugar
2	eggs, beaten
I	teaspoon vanilla extract
¾	cup all-purpose flour
½	teaspoon baking powder
¼	teaspoon sea salt or kosher salt (optional)
3	tablespoons unsweetened cocoa

In the mixing bowl, using an electric mixer on medium speed, cream butter and cream cheese together, gradually add sugar, and continue beating until light and fluffy. Add eggs and vanilla, and continue to beat to a light froth.

In a separate mixing bowl, combine flour, baking powder and salt; add to butter/cream cheese mixture, beating well.

Divide batter into 2 separate mixing bowls, sift cocoa over half of the batter and fold in gently.

Spoon the cocoa batter into the large skillet or 13-inch chef pan. Pour remaining half vanilla batter over cocoa batter. Gently cut threw batter with a butter knife to create a swirling marble effect. Cover, close the vent, and bake on top of the stove over medium-low heat for 20 minutes, test with toothpick.

To serve, allow brownies to cool, and then cut into 2-inch x I ¼-inch bars, serve warm with vanilla ice cream.

Nutritional breakdown does not include ice cream.

NUTRITIONAL BREAKDOWN PER SERVING: Calories 57; Fat Grams 2; Carbohydrate Grams 9; Protein Grams I; Cholesterol mg 2; Sodium mg 74.

THE POINT SYSTEM: Calorie Points I; Protein Points 0; Fat Grams 2; Sodium Points 3; Fiber Points 0; Carbohydrate Points ½; Cholesterol Points 0.

Poppy Seed Icebox Cookies

Yields: 64 cookies
Preparation Time: 1 hour
Equipment: stainless mixing bowls, electric mixer, 12-inch electric skillet, French chef knife

⅓	cup margarine or unsalted butter, softened
⅔	cup sugar
1	egg or 2 egg whites
2	tablespoons skim milk
½	teaspoon almond extract
1¾	cups all-purpose flour
½	teaspoon baking soda
¼	teaspoon salt
¼	teaspoon ground nutmeg
2	tablespoons poppy seeds

In the mixing bowl, using an electric mixer on medium speed, cream margarine or butter, and gradually add sugar, until light and fluffy. Add egg, skim milk and almond extract and continue to beat to a light froth.

In a separate mixing bowl, combine flour, baking soda and nutmeg; add to creamed mixture, beating until ingredients are thoroughly combined. Using a spatula or large spoon, stir in poppy seeds.

Divide dough into 4 equal portions; place each portion on a sheet of plastic wrap, and shape into a 4-inch x 2-inch (10 cm x 5 cm) log. Refrigerate or freeze until firm. Unwrap logs, and cut into ¼-inch (75 mm) slices.

Preheat 12-inch electric skillet or 13-inch chef pan to 275°F (135°C). Place slices 1-inch (2.5 cm) apart. Cover with vent open and cook 20 minutes. Cool on wire racks and serve.

NUTRITIONAL BREAKDOWN PER SERVING: Calories 25; Fat Grams 1; Carbohydrate Grams 5; Protein Grams 0; Cholesterol mg 0; Sodium mg 24.

THE POINT SYSTEM: Calorie Points ½; Protein Points 0; Fat Grams 1; Sodium Points 1; Fiber Points 0; Carbohydrate Points ½; Cholesterol Points 0.

Light Cheesecake

Serves: 12 to 14
Preparation Time: 1 hour 30 minutes
Equipment: Kitchen Machine food cutter, small stainless mixing bowl, large stainless mixing
bowl, electric mixer, 10-inch chef pan

CRUST
⅔   cup graham crackers, grated blade #1
1   tablespoon sifted powdered sugar
1   tablespoon fresh lemon zest, grated blade #1
2   tablespoons margarine or unsalted butter, melted

FILLING
1   15 ounce (430 g) carton low-fat ricotta cheese
1   8 ounce (230 g) package light cream cheese, softened
1   cup sugar or sugar substitute
2   tablespoons all-purpose flour
1   tablespoon fresh lemon zest, grated blade #1
1   tablespoon fresh squeezed lemon juice
2   teaspoons vanilla
2   eggs
2   egg whites
1   8 ounce (230 g) carton plain low-fat yogurt

For crust; in the mixing bowl, combine crackers, powdered sugar and lemon zest with butter or margarine. Mix well, and press into the bottom of 10-inch chef pan or large skillet. Cook over low heat 5 minutes. Set aside to cool.

For filling; in the large mixing bowl, using the electric mixer on medium speed, combine ricotta and cream cheese, sugar, flour, lemon zest, lemon juice and vanilla. Add eggs and egg whites, beating on low speed just until combined. Stir in yogurt. Pour mixture into crust-line pan. Bake over low heat 1 hour 15 minutes or until center appears nearly set when shaken. Cover the pan, close the vent, and chill thoroughly in the refrigerator.

To serve, top with fresh strawberries (optional) or any other fresh fruit.

Nutritional breakdown does not include strawberries

NUTRITIONAL BREAKDOWN PER SERVING: Calories 176; Fat Grams 3; Carbohydrate Grams 26; Protein Grams 9; Cholesterol mg 39; Sodium mg 344.

THE POINT SYSTEM: Calorie Points 2½; Protein Points 1; Fat Grams 3; Sodium Points 15; Fiber Points 0; Carbohydrate Points 1½; Cholesterol Points 4.

Angel Food Cake

On Top of the Stove
Serves: 10
Preparation Time: 2 hours
Equipment: large stainless mixing bowl, electric mixer, mixing bowl, 6-quart stockpot,
4.5-quart Dutch oven cover

1¼	cups (300 ml) egg whites (approximately 7 large eggs)
½	teaspoon salt
1	teaspoon cream of tartar
2	tablespoons water
1½	cups sugar
½	teaspoon vanilla
½	teaspoon almond extract
1	cup cake flour

In the large mixing bowl, using the electric mixer, beat eggs whites and salt at high speed until frothy, about 1 minute. Add cream of tartar, and beat 3 minutes, add water, and continue beating at high speed until egg white stand at peaks, about 3-4 minutes. Turn mixer to low speed; add sugar gradually and flavoring. Beat about ½ minute longer. Sift flour twice, using spatula fold flour into egg whites until mixed thoroughly.

Place an Angel Food Cake tube in center of 6-quart (6 L) stockpot (or make one using a slim, tall, heavy glass inverted). Pour batter into dry pan. Cover with 4.5-quart Dutch oven cover, or 10-inch chef pan inverted on 6-quart, and place on cold, small burner. Turn heat to low. Bake for 50 minutes. DON'T PEEK! LIFTING THE COVER WILL CAUSE CAKE TO FALL. Cake top will cook dry but not brown.

To cool, place four knife handles evenly under edges of inverted pan. Let cool for 1 hour, and then remove cake. Loosen with knife around edge of glass, and lightly brush off crumbs.

Serve with Almond Sauce, Chocolate-Marshmallow Sauce or Red Plum Sauce, pages 187 and 188.

NUTRITIONAL BREAKDOWN PER SERVING: Calories 150; Fat Grams 0; Carbohydrate Grams 34; Protein Grams 0; Cholesterol mg 0; Sodium mg 300.

THE POINT SYSTEM: Calorie Points 2; Protein Points 0; Fat Grams 0; Sodium Points 13; Fiber Points 0; Carbohydrate Points 2; Cholesterol Points 0.

Almond Sauce

Yield: ¾ cup
Preparation Time: 15 minutes
Equipment: 1-quart saucepan

3	tablespoons sugar
2	teaspoons cornstarch
½	cup (120 ml) water
3	tablespoons Amaretto
½	teaspoon fresh squeezed lemon juice
2	tablespoons sliced almonds
¼	teaspoon almond extract

In 1-quart (1.5 L) saucepan, combine sugar and cornstarch, and stir in water. Place over medium heat and bring to a simmer. Cook 2 minutes or until thickened, stirring constantly.

Stir in Amaretto and lemon juice, heat until mixture comes to a simmer. Remove from heat and stir in almonds and extract.

NUTRITIONAL BREAKDOWN PER SERVING: Calories 65; Fat Grams 2; Carbohydrate Grams 11; Protein Grams 1; Cholesterol mg 0; Sodium mg 1; Calorie Points 1.

Chocolate Marshmallow Sauce

Yields: 1 cup
Preparation Time: 15 minutes
Equipment: 1-quart (1.5 L) saucepan

⅓	cup miniature marshmallows
2	tablespoons unsweetened cocoa
1	tablespoon cornstarch
1	cup (240 ml) skim milk
1	tablespoon light corn syrup
1	teaspoon vanilla extract
¼	teaspoon ground cinnamon
¼	cup miniature marshmallows
1	tablespoon chopped pecans

In the 1-quart (1.5 L) saucepan, combine ⅓ cup marshmallows, cocoa, and cornstarch over medium heat. Gradually add milk and corn syrup, stirring constantly until thickened. Remove from heat, stir in vanilla, cinnamon, ¼ cup marshmallows and pecans.

NUTRITIONAL BREAKDOWN PER SERVING: Calories 84; Fat Grams 1 ½; Carbohydrate Grams 19; Protein Grams 0; Cholesterol mg 0; Sodium mg 2; Calorie Points 1.

Red Plum Sauce

Yields: 1¼ cups
Preparation Time: 15 minutes
Equipment: 2-quart saucepan

½	cup sugar
2	teaspoons cornstarch
½	teaspoon ground cinnamon
½	cup (120 ml) peach or apricot nectar
1	cup sliced red fresh plums, pit removed
½	teaspoon almond extract

In the 2-quart (2 L) saucepan, combine sugar, cornstarch and cinnamon, over medium heat, stir well. Add nectar, and continue to stir until smooth. Add plums and bring to a simmer, stirring constantly. Remove from heat and stir in almond extract.

NUTRITIONAL BREAKDOWN PER SERVING: Calories 74; Fat Grams 0; Carbohydrate Grams 19; Protein Grams 0; Cholesterol mg 0; Sodium mg 2; Calorie Points 1.

Stovetop Strawberry Shortcake

Serves: 8

Preparation Time: 30 minutes

Equipment: 13-inch chef pan or 12-inch electric skillet, medium stainless mixing bowl

	Baking mix
4	cups strawberries
¼	cup sugar
	Non-dairy whipped topping or whipped cream

Prepare shortcake recipe according to directions on box, adding additional sugar. Roll dough out to ½-inch (1.5 cm) thickness; using a 3-inch (7.5 cm) diameter cookie cutter cut out shortcake rounds.

Preheat 13-inch chef pan or 12-inch electric skillet over medium heat 275°F (135°C). Place shortcake in pan, cover, open vent open, and bake for 20 minutes. DO NOT PEEK. After cooling, cut shortcakes in half lengthwise.

While shortcakes are baking, remove stems from strawberries, wash and cut in half. Place in medium mixing bowl and sprinkle with sugar. Let set until shortcakes are cooled.

To serve, place bottom half of shortcake on individual dessert plates, spoon 2-3 tablespoons strawberries onto shortcake, place top half of shortcake on top of strawberries, spoon on more strawberries and top with whipped cream.

NUTRITIONAL BREAKDOWN PER SERVING: Calories 296; Fat Grams 10; Carbohydrate Grams 50; Protein Grams 3; Cholesterol mg 0; Sodium mg 307.

THE POINT SYSTEM: Calorie Points 4; Protein Points 0; Fat Grams 10; Sodium Points 13; Fiber Points 1; Carbohydrate Points 3½; Cholesterol Points 0.

Fresh Strawberry Trifle

Serves: 8
Preparation Time: 2 hours 30 minutes
Equipment: 2 quart saucepan, small stainless mixing bowl

2	cups (480 ml) skim milk, divided
1	egg, beaten
3	tablespoons cornstarch
2	tablespoons honey
1	teaspoon vanilla extract
½	teaspoon orange extract
6	Angel Food cake slices, see recipe page 186, or ladyfingers sliced lengthwise
1	tablespoon Triple Sec
3	cups fresh strawberries, trimmed, sliced and divided

With a serrated knife, slice Angel Food cake to create 6 equal cake rounds. Trim cakes to size of Trifle dish or clear glass serving bowl leaving about ¼-inch clearance around edges.

CUSTARD FILLING

Combine 1¾ cups (420 ml) milk with beaten egg in 2 quart (2 L) saucepan. Beat with a wire whisk 1 to 2 minutes or until foamy.

In the small mixing bowl combine remaining ¼ cup (60 ml) milk with cornstarch, stir until smooth, add honey and stir well. Add to milk and egg mixture, and cook over medium heat, stirring constantly until thickened. Remove from heat and stir in vanilla and orange extract. Cover and chill.

ASSEMBLY

Place a cake slice on bottom of trifle dish or clear bowl. Sprinkle with Triple Sec, and arrange ⅓ cup sliced strawberries on top of each cake. Top the three cake/strawberry layers with half of chilled custard. Repeat with three layers of cake and strawberries. Top with remaining custard. Cover and chill at least 2 hours.

To serve, garnish with whole strawberries and mint leaves.

NUTRITIONAL BREAKDOWN PER SERVING: Calories 232; Fat Grams 1; Carbohydrate Grams 48; Protein Grams 7; Cholesterol mg 37; Sodium mg 309.

THE POINT SYSTEM: Calorie Points 3; Protein Points 1; Fat Grams 1; Sodium Points 13; Fiber Points 1; Carbohydrate Points 3; Cholesterol Points 4.

Raspberry Mash

Serves: 8
Preparation Time: 3 hours
Equipment: 10-inch chef pan or large skillet, 2-quart (2 L) saucepan,
Electric Mixer, large stainless mixing bowl,

3	tablespoons reduced calorie margarine or unsalted butter
2	cups crushed vanilla wafers
1	16 ounce (460 g) bag frozen raspberries, thawed, or 1 pound fresh
⅓	cup sugar
⅓	cup (80 ml) skim milk
2	egg yolks, beaten
1	envelope unflavored gelatin
½	teaspoon vanilla extract
¼	teaspoon salt
2	egg whites
¼	teaspoon cream of tartar
2	tablespoons sugar
	Fresh raspberries mint for garnish

To create the crust, in the 10-inch chef pan or large skillet, melt butter over low heat. Add crushed wafers, stirring well. With a potato masher or pancake spatula, press mixture evenly over bottom of pan. Cook over low heat for 10 minutes, and set aside.

In the 2-quart (2 L) saucepan, mash raspberries with potato masher, add ½ cup sugar, skim milk, egg yolks, gelatin, vanilla and salt. Mix well, cover, open vent, and cook over medium heat until mixture simmers, stirring occasionally. Let stand for 30-40 minutes or until mixture thickens slightly, or place in refrigerator to cool.

In the mixing bowl, beat the egg whites and cream of tartar with the electric mixer at high speed until foamy. Gradually add 2 tablespoons sugar, beating until peaks form to make a meringue. Gently fold raspberry mixture into egg whites, pour over crust and chill 2 hours until firm.

To serve, slice into 8 equal portions, remove to dessert plates, and garnish with fresh raspberries and mint leaves.

NUTRITIONAL BREAKDOWN PER SERVING: Calories 292; Fat Grams 7; Carbohydrate Grams 45; Protein Grams 13; Cholesterol mg 69; Sodium mg 140.

THE POINT SYSTEM: Calorie Points 4; Protein Points 2; Fat Grams 7; Sodium Points 6; Fiber Points 1; Carbohydrate Points 3; Cholesterol Points 7.

Baked Apples

Serves: 5
Preparation Time: 50 minutes
Equipment: paring knife, 4-quart stockpot, I-quart saucepan

5	whole apples, washed and cores removed
I	tablespoon raw sugar
¼	teaspoon cinnamon
4	tablespoons unsalted butter
I	cup sugar
I	tablespoon water
	Raisins and sliced almonds for garnish

Pare the apples by peeling about ½-inch of skin around the center, leaving skin on top and bottom.

Place apples in the 4-quart (4 L) stockpot, sprinkle sugar and cinnamon on the top of the apple where the stem was removed, cover, close vent, and cook the waterless way over low heat 20-25 minutes.

In the I-quart (1.5 L) saucepan, make syrup, over medium heat with butter, sugar and water, stir as cooking. About 4 to 5 minutes.

To serve, place apples in individual serving bowls, top with syrup, sliced almonds and raisins.

NUTRITIONAL BREAKDOWN PER SERVING: Calories 199; Fat Grams 5; Carbohydrate Grams 41; Protein Grams 0; Cholesterol mg 12; Sodium mg 48.

THE POINT SYSTEM: Calorie Points 2½; Protein Points 0; Fat Grams 5; Sodium Points 2; Fiber Points 1½; Carbohydrate Points 3; Cholesterol Points 1.

Chocolate Mousse

Serves: 6
Preparation Time: 30 minutes
Equipment: French chef knife, cutting board, 11-inch wok/saucier,
medium stainless mixing bowl, electric mixer

6	ounces (170 g) semi-sweet chocolate, chopped into small pieces
⅓	cup (80 ml) water
1	tablespoon unsalted butter, softened
2	tablespoons rum
3	3 eggs, separated
	Mint leaves and fresh berries for garnish

In the 11-inch wok/saucier, combine chocolate with water, cook over low heat so the chocolate and water form a thick cream, remove from heat and allow to cool slightly. Whisk in softened butter, add the rum and whisk in egg yolks one at a time. Set aside to cool.

In the mixing bowl, with the electric mixer, beat egg whites until stiff. Gently fold into cooled chocolate sauce. Pour into individual martini glasses or custard cups and chill overnight or 2-3 hours before serving.

To serve, top with mint leaves and fresh berries.

NUTRITIONAL BREAKDOWN PER SERVING: Calories 189; Fat Grams 12; Carbohydrate Grams 19; Protein Grams 3; Cholesterol mg 112; Sodium mg 24.

THE POINT SYSTEM: Calorie Points 2½; Protein Points 0; Fat Grams 12; Sodium Points 1; Fiber Points 0; Carbohydrate Points 1; Cholesterol Points 5.

Banana Chiffon Cake

Serves: 12
Preparation Time: 1 hour 15 minutes
Equipment: 2 large stainless mixing bowl, electric mixer,
6-quart (6 L) stockpot, 4½ Dutch oven cover.

2	cups cake flour
1½	cups sugar
1	tablespoon baking powder
1	teaspoon salt
½	cup (120 ml) canola oil
1½	cups (360 ml) egg substitute (or 1 egg yolk)
¾	cup (180 ml) water
1	ripe banana, mashed
1	teaspoon vanilla
6	egg whites
½	teaspoon cream of tartar

GLAZE

Powdered sugar
Water
Bananas, sliced for garnish

In the large mixing bowl, sift together cake flour, baking powder and salt. Add oil, egg substitute, and water. Mix well with electric mixer. Add banana and vanilla, beat well.

In the other mixing bowl, whip egg whites and cream of tartar to form airy stiff peaks. Gently fold banana cake batter into egg whites.

In the 6-quart Stockpot, make a tube pan by placing a tall thick glass inverted into the center of the pan. Spray the pan and glass with a cooking spray. Pour cake batter around the glass, cover with 4½-quart Dutch oven cover. Bake over medium heat for 5 minutes, reduce heat to low, and continue baking 45-50 minutes. Remove from heat, allow to cool, 30-40 minutes. Run a knife around edges and center glass, invert pan onto cake plate.

Alternative, preheat oven to 350°F (180°C), lightly coat Bundt cake pan with cooking spray, pour cake batter into pan and bake 45-55 minutes, invert to cool.

To serve, glaze with thin icing of powdered sugar and water combined. Top with sliced bananas.

NUTRITIONAL BREAKDOWN PER SERVING: Calories 267; Fat Grams 10; Carbohydrate Grams 42; Protein Grams 4; Cholesterol mg 18; Sodium mg 279.

THE POINT SYSTEM: Calorie Points 3½; Protein Points 0; Fat Grams 10; Sodium Points 12; Fiber Points 0; Carbohydrate Points 2½; Cholesterol Points 2.

Pineapple Upside-Down Cake

Serves: 12
Preparation Time: 35 minutes
Equipment: large stainless mixing bowl, electric mixer, large skillet

1	20 ounce (570 g) can sliced pineapple (reserve liquid)
1	box pineapple upside down cake mix, or yellow, orange or lemon cake mix
3	eggs
¼	stick unsalted butter, or cooking spray
½	cup raw sugar
8	maraschino cherries

Drain pineapple juice into measuring cup. In the mixing bowl, using the electric mixer, combine cake mix, ½ cup pineapple juice, and eggs, mix well.

In the large skillet, melt the butter over low heat, turning to coat the skillet up the sides to near the rim. Allow skillet to cool slightly, dust bottom and sides with sugar. Drain pineapple rings on paper towels and place in the bottom of skillet, and place a maraschino cherry in the center of each pineapple ring. Pour cake batter into the Skillet.

Cover, close the vent, and cook over medium heat 5 minutes, reduce the heat to low and cook for 25-30 minutes. Test for doneness with toothpick. Invert large cake plate over skillet, turn quickly and lift skillet from cake.

To serve, with a serrated knife, slice into 12 equal servings. Serve warm of cold.

NUTRITIONAL BREAKDOWN PER SERVING: Calories 247; Fat Grams 9; Carbohydrate Grams 40; Protein Grams 2; Cholesterol mg 38; Sodium mg 257.

THE POINT SYSTEM: Calorie Points 3½; Protein Points 0; Fat Grams 9; Sodium Points 11; Fiber Points 0; Carbohydrate Points 2½; Cholesterol Points 4.

Variation, from scratch

Apricot Upside-Down Cake

Serves: 12
Preparation Time: 1 hour
Equipment: large skillet, large mixing bowl, electric mixer

1	stick, margarine or unsalted butter
1	cup light brown sugar
2	14.5 ounce (410 g) cans apricot halves, drained and juice reserved
1	8 ounce (230 g) can crushed pineapple, drained and juice reserved
1	teaspoon cinnamon
½	teaspoon nutmeg
1	stick (115 g) unsalted butter or margarine
1	cup sugar
2	eggs
1	cup flour, sifted
1½	teaspoon baking powder
½	teaspoon baking soda
½	teaspoon salt
½	cup (120 ml) buttermilk
1	teaspoon vanilla

In the large skillet, melt butter, turning to coat the sides of the pan. Add brown sugar and ½ cup (120 ml) apricot juice to butter. Simmer about 5 minutes or until slightly thickened. Arrange apricot halves in pan; sprinkle crushed pineapple over apricots, sprinkle with cinnamon and nutmeg. Remove from heat and set aside.

In the mixing bowl, cream butter and sugar, add eggs, and mix well on medium speed. Alternately add flour, baking powder, baking soda and buttermilk, mix well. Add vanilla last. Pour batter over fruit mixture. Cover, close the vent, and cook over low heat 45 minutes. Cool slightly.

To serve, invert onto cake plate and serve warm with vanilla ice cream.

Carrot Cake with Cream Cheese Frosting

Serves: 16

Preparation Time: 1 hour

Equipment: Kitchen Machine food cutter, large mixing bowl, electric mixer, large skillet

CARROT CAKE

1¾	cup all-purpose flour
1¾	cup sugar
½	cup oat or wheat bran
1	teaspoon baking powder
1	teaspoon baking soda
1	teaspoon cinnamon
3	cups carrots, shredded blade #1
⅔	cup (160 ml) oil or applesauce
3	egg whites
¼	cup (60 ml) corn syrup

Coat Large Skillet with cooking spray…

Combine flour, sugar, oat or wheat bran, baking powder, baking soda, and cinnamon. Add grated carrots, cooking oil (or applesauce), egg whites, and corn syrup. Beat with electric mixer until thoroughly mixed. Pour batter into large skillet, cover, close the vent, and bake on top of the stove on low heat for 45-55 minutes. Test for doneness with a toothpick. To remove cake from pan, shake the skillet to loosen from sides and bottom, invert over cake plate. Allow to cool slightly before frosting.

CREAM CHEESE FROSTING

½	cup fat-free cream cheese
3¼	cups powdered sugar, separated
2	teaspoons vanilla
½	teaspoon fresh lemon zest, grated blade #1 (or orange zest)

In a mixing bowl, using the electric mixer at medium speed, combine cream cheese, 2 cups powdered sugar, vanilla and lemon zest, mix well. When thoroughly combined, gradually add the remaining 1¼ cups of powdered sugar until consistency for spreading.

To serve, frost carrot cake, sprinkle with shredded carrots and top with mint leaves. Serve warm or cold.

NUTRITIONAL BREAKDOWN PER SERVING: Calories 338; Fat Grams 9; Carbohydrate Grams 63; Protein Grams 3; Cholesterol mg 1; Sodium mg 158.

THE POINT SYSTEM: Calorie Points 5; Protein Points 0; Fat Grams 9; Sodium Points 7; Fiber Points 0; Carbohydrate Points 4; Cholesterol Points 0.

Chocolate Chip Cookie Bars

Yields: 24

Preparation Time: 40 minutes

Equipment: large stainless mixing bowl, electric mixer, medium mixing bowl, 13-inch chef pan

1	cup low fat margarine or unsalted butter
1¾	cups brown sugar, packed
2	eggs
1	teaspoon vanilla
1	teaspoon baking soda
½	teaspoon salt
2	cups rolled oats
2¼	cups all-purpose flour
1	12 ounce (345 g) bag chocolate chips

In a mixing bowl, using the electric mixer, cream butter or margarine together with sugar, add eggs and vanilla and blend gently or low speed.

In the medium mixing bowl, combine baking soda, salt, rolled oats and flour. Slowly add the flour mixture to the butter mixture and blend thoroughly. Stir in the chocolate chips with a spatula to combine.

Press the chocolate chip mixture into a cold chef pan or large skillet. Cover, close the vent, and cook over medium heat for 5 minutes, reduce to low and cook 25-30 minutes. Test for doneness with a toothpick, and allow to rest 5-10 minutes before cutting and serving.

NUTRITIONAL BREAKDOWN PER SERVING: Calories 217; Fat Grams 8; Carbohydrate Grams 36; Protein Grams 3; Cholesterol mg 0; Sodium mg 195.

THE POINT SYSTEM: Calorie Points 3; Protein Points 0; Fat Grams 8; Sodium Points 8; Fiber Points 0; Carbohydrate Points 2½; Cholesterol Points 0.

Rice Pudding

Serves: 4
Preparation Time: 30 minutes
Equipment: 3-quart (3 L) saucepan, small stainless mixing bowl

I	cup rice, washed and drained
I½	cups (360 ml) milk
I	vanilla bean
	Pinch of salt
	Raisins (optional)
½	cup sugar
I	egg, beaten
	Mint leaves for garnish

Place rice in 3-quart (3 L) saucepan, add enough water to cover rice, cover, open the vent, and bring to a boil over medium-high heat. As soon as the water has been absorbed (about 10 minutes), add milk, vanilla bean, and salt. Raisins can be added if desired. Cover, close the vent, and reduce the heat to medium-low, cook for 10 minutes. Remove from heat.

In the mixing bowl, combine the sugar and beaten egg, mix well. Add to rice mixture, mixing thoroughly. Cover, close the vent, and let stand to finish cooking, about 5-10 minutes.

To serve, top with whipped cream (optional), and garnish with mint leaves. Serve warm or chilled.

NUTRITIONAL BREAKDOWN PER SERVING: Calories 187; Fat Grams 0; Carbohydrate Grams 41; Protein Grams 5; Cholesterol mg 2; Sodium mg 62.

THE POINT SYSTEM: Calorie Points 2½; Protein Points 1; Fat Grams 0; Sodium Points 3; Fiber Points 0; Carbohydrate Points 2½; Cholesterol Points 0.

Caramel Flan

Serves: 8
Preparation Time: 3 hours
Equipment: 1-quart saucepan, thermo server/double boiler, large stainless mixing bowl,
electric mixer, large skillet, steamer rack, 4½-quart Dutch oven cover

CARAMEL

½	cup sugar
¼	cup (60 ml) water

CUSTARD

4	eggs, slightly beaten
6	tablespoon sugar
2	cups (480 ml) half-n-half (half milk, half cream)
1	teaspoon vanilla
1	cup (240 ml) water

To make the Caramel; in the 1-quart (1.5 L) saucepan, combine sugar and water, cook over low heat and stir until sugar is completely dissolved. When completely dissolved, increase to high heat, continuing to stir until syrup turns a deep golden brown color. Remove from heat and pour into thermo server/double boiler pan. Turn pan to coat the bottom and sides.

To make the Custard; in the large mixing bowl, using the electric mixer on low speed, combine the eggs, sugar, half-n-half, vanilla, and water, mix well. Pour custard mixture into Caramelized thermo server/double boiler pan and cover tightly with aluminum foil.

To the large skillet, add 2 cups (480 ml) water. Set the steamer rack on the skillet, place the double boiler on the steamer rack, and cover with 4½-quart Dutch oven cover. Turn to medium-high heat and form the vapor seal, reduce heat to medium-low, and cook for 45 minutes. Remove from heat, remove aluminum foil, and allow to cool 15-20 minutes. Refrigerate for 1-2 hours before serving.

To serve, place a serving dish over the double boiler (large enough to accommodate the caramel sauce), invert to serving dish. Garnish with orange or lemon zest.

NUTRITIONAL BREAKDOWN PER SERVING: Calories 174; Fat Grams 7; Carbohydrate Grams 25; Protein Grams 4; Cholesterol mg 22; Sodium mg 52.

THE POINT SYSTEM: Calorie Points 2½; Protein Points 0; Fat Grams 7; Sodium Points 2; Fiber Points 0; Carbohydrate Points 1½; Cholesterol Points 2.

Bread Pudding

Serves: 8

Preparation Time: 30 minutes

Equipment: Kitchen Machine food cutter, 13-inch chef pan, 3-quart saucepan,
large stainless mixing bowl

4	1-inch (2.5 cm) slice French, Cuban or Italian bread, cubed
2	cups (480 ml) skim milk
½	cup brown sugar
1	tablespoon unsalted butter
½	cup raisins
3	eggs, lightly beaten
1	teaspoon cinnamon
½	teaspoon salt
½	teaspoon vanilla
2	teaspoons orange zest, grated blade #1
2	cups (480 ml) water

In the 13-inch (33 cm) chef pan, dry bread cubes in low temperature oven 200°F (90°C) for 20 minutes, or dry overnight at room temperature.

In the 3-quart (3 L) saucepan, heat milk, sugar, butter and raisins over low heat.

In the large mixing bowl, whisk together, eggs, cinnamon, salt, vanilla, and orange zest. Whisk in hot milk mixture, and add bread cubes. Stir for 15-20 seconds, pushing floating bread cubes into mixture. Do not stir longer or bread will become too soft.

Pour mixture back into 3-quart (3 L) saucepan, cover, close the vent, and cook over medium heat for 5 minutes, reduce to low heat and continue to cook for 30 minutes.

To serve, top with Rum or Piňa Colada Sauce, recipe and nutritional breakdown page 202

Rum Sauce

1	stick (115 g) unsalted butter
½	cup raw sugar
¼	cup (60 ml) dark rum

Melt butter in 1-quart (1.5 L) saucepan, add sugar and cook 5 minutes over medium heat, stirring constantly. Remove from heat, add rum, return to heat and cook for 1-2 minutes.

To serve, allow to cool slightly, pour over top of Bread Pudding and garnish with orange zest.

Pina Colada Sauce

1	stick (115 g) unsalted butter
½	cup raw sugar
1	teaspoon pineapple extract
¼	cup fresh grated coconut, blade #1 Kitchen Machine
½	cup canned or fresh pineapple chunks

Melt butter in 1-quart (1.5 L) saucepan, add sugar, pineapple extract, coconut, pineapple chunks, and cook 5 minutes over medium heat, stirring constantly.

To serve, allow to cool slightly, pour over top of Bread Pudding and garnish with mint leaves.

NUTRITIONAL BREAKDOWN PER SERVING: Calories 137; Fat Grams 2; Carbohydrate Grams 26; Protein Grams 5; Cholesterol mg 5; Sodium mg 147.

THE POINT SYSTEM: Calorie Points 2; Protein Points ½; Fat Grams 2; Sodium Points 6; Fiber Points 0; Carbohydrate Points 1½; Cholesterol Points 0.

Easy One-Egg Cake

Serves: 12
Preparation Time: 30 minutes
Equipment: 3-quart saucepan, large stainless mixing bowl, electric mixer

Unsalted butter or non-stick cooking spray
1¼ cups un-sifted all-purpose flour
¼ cup sugar
2 teaspoons baking powder
½ teaspoon salt
¼ cup shortening
⅔ cup (160 ml) skim milk
1 egg
1 teaspoon vanilla
1 Hershey's dark chocolate candy bar*

In the mixing bowl, using the electric mixing on low speed, combine flour, sugar, baking powder, salt, shortening, milk, about 1-2 minutes. Add egg and vanilla, mix well on medium speed, about 1-2 minutes.

Generously butter the 3-quart saucepan, and pour batter into pan. Cover, close the vent, and bake over low heat 18-20 minutes.

To serve, invert hot cake onto serving plate, top with candy bar to melt and spread with a butter knife or spatula to coat. Top with chocolate covered strawberries, see recipe page 181.

NUTRITIONAL BREAKDOWN PER SERVING: Calories 142; Fat Grams 4; Carbohydrate Grams 23; Protein Grams 2; Cholesterol mg 0; Sodium mg 149.

THE POINT SYSTEM: Calorie Points 2; Protein Points 0; Fat Grams 4; Sodium Points 7; Fiber Points 0; Carbohydrate Points 1½; Cholesterol Points 0.

*For nutritional breakdown on chocolate bar refer to wrapper.

Spice Mixtures

GARAM MASALA

1	bay leaf
½	teaspoon whole black pepper
½	teaspoon whole cloves
½	teaspoon cinnamon stick
½	teaspoon cardamom

Garam Masala is simply a blend of fresh roasted spices. In the 7-inch chef pan, individually dry roast each spice over medium heat until fragrant. Using a coffee grinder (used for spices only) or a mortar and pestle, grind spices together.

INDIAN CURRY SPICE MIX

½	cup coriander seeds
¼	cup cumin seeds
8	dried red chilies, seeded
1	tablespoon peppercorns
1	tablespoon black mustard seeds
2	tablespoons turmeric
2	tablespoons fenugreek

In the 7-inch Chef Pan, individually dry roast each spice over medium heat until fragrant. Using a coffee grinder (used for spices only) or a mortar and pestle, grind spices together. Store spice mixture in a covered jar in a dark place, DO NOT keep in refrigerator and it will keep approximately 3 months.

5-SPICE MIX

1	tablespoon whole fennel seed
1	tablespoon star anise
1	cinnamon stick
1	tablespoon whole cloves
1	tablespoon Szechuan pepper corns

In the 8-inch chef pan or small skillet, dry roast one spice at a time until aromatic. Grind in spice grinder or use a mortar and pestle.

ROATED RICE POWDER

Heat 8-inch chef pan or small skillet over medium high heat, add ¼ cup raw rice, preferably glutinous rice, and stir constantly as rice heats. After several minutes it will have a lightly toasted aroma and will begin to turn pale brown. Keep stirring until all the rice has changed to a light tan color, then transfer to a spice grinder or large mortar and pestle and grind to a fine powder.

Roasted rice powder keeps well in a sealed glass jar for several months. Use as needed in Thai and Vietnamese dishes.

BOUQUET GARNI
Equal portions of:
Dried dill weed
Thyme
Basil
Parsley
Marjoram
Tarragon

Variation of Bouquet Garni, a mixture of herbs (tied by the stems or placed in a cloth bag,) to flavor broth or stew and then removed before serving.

Traditional Bouquet Garni includes fresh parsley, fresh thyme and dried bay leaf, tied together in a bundle.

TAHINI

Tahini is available in Middle Eastern and some health food stores. You can prepare your own by grinding sesame seeds and adding enough sesame oil to give the mixture the consistency of peanut butter.

BLANCHED ALMONDS

Cover almonds with 1 cup water, bring to a boil, turn off heat, and soak overnight (at least 4 to 5 hours.) Drain, peel outer skin, and slice lengthwise.

INDEX

5-Spice Mix.................................. 205

Almond Sauce.............................. 187

Angel Food Cake........................... 186

Appetizers

    Hot Crab Dip.......................... 77

    Roasted Pepper Salad................. 62

    Sesame Chicken Wings................ 79

    Wrapped Chestnuts................... 78

Apple(s)

    Apple-Chicken Rolls................. 123

    Apricot Apple Chutney............... 75

    Baked Apples....................... 192

Apricot Apple Chutney..................... 75

Apricot Up-Side Down Cake................. 196

Artichokes, Stuffed....................... 160

Asparagus

    Asparagus Mushroom Sauté........... 153

    Orange Roughy a la Asparagus....... 125

Avocado

    Guacamole........................... 101

Baby Back Ribs............................ 98

Baked Apples.............................. 192

Banana Chiffon Cake....................... 194

Bars, Chocolate Chip Cookies.............. 198

Basic Crepes.............................. 141

Basic Lasagna............................. 96

Basmati Pea Pilaf......................... 168

BBQ

    Baby Back Ribs...................... 98

    Catfish Barbecue.................... 129

Bean(s)

    Green Bean and Fennel Salad........ 68

    Pinto Bean Soup..................... 61

Beef

    Basic Lasagna....................... 96

    Beef and Chinese Vegetables......... 86

    Beef Fajitas........................ 99

    Beef with Broccoli.................. 84

    Blarney Stone Stew.................. 93

    Boeuf Bourguinon.................... 82

    Chinese Beef-Noodle Soup............ 59

    Griddle Kabobs...................... 85

    Ground Beef Skillet Casserole....... 91

    Italian Meat Balls.................. 90

    Marinated Flank Steak............... 94

    Meatballs a la Swiss................ 89

    Meatloaf............................ 95

    Meat Sauce.......................... 97

    Saucy Beef and Noodles.............. 83

    Stuffed Peppers..................... 104

    Swedish Meatballs................... 88

    Thai Grilled Sirloin Salad.......... 53

    Wedding Soup........................ 56

Blanched Almonds.......................... 205

Blarney Stone Stew........................ 93

Blintzes, Strawberry Cheese............... 141

Bouquet Garni............................. 205

Bourguignon, Beoeuf....................... 82

Bow, Hom.................................. 169

Bread

    Bread Pudding....................... 201

    Cornbread........................... 164

    Garlic Bread........................ 179

    Griddle Oat Scones.................. 166

    Hom Bow............................. 169

    Homemade Croutons................... 70

Italian Focaccia............................. 163

Nan Bread................................. 167

Soda Bread................................ 179

Breakfast Burritos............................. 145

Broccoli

Beef with Broccoli......................... 84

Turkey with Orzo and Broccoli.......... 122

Vegetable Stir Fry......................... 152

Brownies, Marbled............................. 183

Burritos, Breakfast............................ 145

Cabbage

Skillet Cabbage............................ 161

Stuffed, Cabbage Rolls.................... 103

Cacciatore, Chicken............................ 112

Caesar Salad and Grilled Chicken................. 65

Cake(s)

Angel Food Cake.......................... 186

Apricot Upside-Down Cake.............. 196

Banana Chiffon Cake...................... 194

Carrot Cake w/ Cream Cheese Frosting 197

Easy One-Egg Cake....................... 203

Fresh Strawberry Trifle................... 190

Light Cheesecake.......................... 185

Pineapple Upside-Down Cake........... 195

Stovetop Strawberry Shortcake........ 189

Caramel Flan.................................. 200

Carbonaro, Pasta.............................. 175

Carrot(s)

Carrot Cake w/ Cream Cheese Frosting 197

Spicy Carrots............................. 151

Vegetable Stir Fry........................ 152

Cashews

Spicy Wehani with Cashews............. 171

Casserole

Egg Casserole............................ 144

Ground Beef Skillet Casserole.......... 91

Catfish Barbecue.............................. 129

Cauliflower

Indian Cauliflower Salad................. 64

Cheese

Cheese Fondue............................ 148

Cream Cheese Frosting.................. 197

Light Cheesecake.......................... 185

Mardi-Gras Family Omelet.............. 143

Cheese

Pasta Carbonaro.......................... 175

Spinach Cheese Jumbo Shells.......... 142

Strawberry Cheese Blintzes............. 141

Chestnuts, Wrapped........................... 78

Chicken

Apple-Chicken Rolls...................... 123

Caesar Salad and Grilled Chicken....... 65

Chicken and Roasted Garlic............. 110

Chicken Cacciatore....................... 112

Chicken Enchiladas....................... 120

Chicken Satay with Peanut Sauce....... 117

Chicken Thighs Marengo................. 114

Chicken Tikka............................. 116

Couscous with Chicken Thighs......... 172

Evening Parmesan Chicken............. 113

Lemon Baked Chicken................... 111

Lemon Sesame Chicken.................. 109

Paella.................................... 133

Roasted Chicken with Rosemary....... 115

Sesame Chicken Wings.................. 79

Teriyaki Chicken......................... 121

Chickpea

Chickpea Soup with Cumin and Cilantro 51

Hummus.................................. 80

Chiffon Cake, Banana......................... 194

Chili, Pork 'n Pineapple....................... 92

Chinese

Beef and Chinese Vegetables........... 86

Chinese Beef-Noodle Soup............. 59

Chinese "Not Fried" Rice............... 173

Chinese Salad............................ 57

Egg Fu Yung............................. 147

INDEX

Chive(s)

    Scallops with Chives and Peppers…..... 126

Chocolate

    Chocolate Chip Cookie Bars………… 198

    Chocolate Glazed Poached Pears……. 181

    Chocolate Marshmallow Sauce……… 187

    Chocolate Mouse…………………….. 193

Chutney, Apricot Apple………………….... 75

Cilantro

    Chickpea Soup with Cumin & Cilantro 51

Clams

    Paella……………………………. 133

Company Tossed Salad…………………… 70

Cookies

    Chocolate Chip Cookie Bars………… 198

    Poppy Seed Ice Box Cookies………... 184

Cornbread………………………………. 165

Couscous with Chicken Thighs………………. 172

Crab

    Hot Crab Dip……………………. 77

    Stuffed Mushrooms…………………. 76

Cream Cheese Frosting…………………… 197

Crepes

    Basic Crepes……………………... 141

    Strawberry Cheese Blintzes…………... 141

Croutons, Homemade…………………….. 70

Cucumber

    Orange Cucumber Salad……………. 55

    Raita……………………………... 69

Cumin

    Chickpea Soup and Cilantro………….. 51

Curry

    Thai Red Curry Shrimp and Pineapple.. 132

    Vegetable Curry……………………. 157

Dessert

    Almond Sauce…………………….... 187

    Angel Food Cake………………….. 186

    Apricot Upside-Down Cake…………. 196

Baked Apples………………………… 192

Banana Chiffon Cake………………… 194

Bread Pudding……………………….. 201

Carmel Flan…………………………... 200

Carrot Cake w/Cream Cheese Frosting 197

Chocolate Chip Cookie Bars………… 198

Chocolate Glazed Poached Pears……. 181

Chocolate-Marshmallow Sauce……… 187

Chocolate Mouse…………………….. 193

Easy One-Egg Cake………………….. 203

Fresh Strawberry Trifle………………. 190

Fruit and Ginger Pears………………... 182

Light Cheesecake……………………... 185

Marbled Brownies……………………. 183

Piña Colada Sauce……………………. 202

Pineapple Upside-Down Cake……….. 195

Poppy Seed Icebox Cookies…………... 184

Raspberry Mash……………………... 191

Red Plum Sauce………………………. 188

Rice Pudding…………………………... 199

Rum Sauce……………………………... 202

Stovetop Strawberry Shortcake…….... 189

Dips

    Guacamole…………………………... 101

    Hot Crab Dip……………………... 77

    Soy Dipping Sauce…………………... 159

Dressings

    French Salad Dressing………………... 72

    Italian Salad Dressing………………... 71

    Shrimp Dressing……………………... 66

    Southwest Vinegar…………………... 73

    Tomato-Herb………………………... 74

Dutch Babies……………………………….... 164

Easy One-Egg Cake……………………….. 203

Rice

    Basmati Pea Pilaf…………………..… 168

    Chinese "Not Fried" Rice…………..… 173

Rice
- Paella..........183
- Rice Pudding..........199
- Spicy Wehani with Cashews..........171

Roasted
- Chicken and Roasted Garlic..........110
- Roasted Chicken with Rosemary..........112
- Roasted Pepper Salad..........62
- Roasted Rice Powder..........205

Rosemary
- Roasted Chicken with Rosemary..........112
- Rosemary Potatoes..........156

Roughy
- Orange Rough a la Asparagus..........125

Rum Sauce..........202

Salad
- Caesar Salad and Grilled Chicken..........65
- Chinese Salad..........57
- Company Tossed Salad..........70
- German Potato Salad..........54
- Green Beans and Fennel Salad..........68
- Indian Cauliflower Salad..........64
- Layer Salad..........58
- Orange Cucumber Salad..........55
- Pasta Shrimp Salad..........176
- Patata-Piccata Salad..........67
- Poppy Seed Fruit Salad..........52
- Potato Salad..........173
- Roasted Pepper Salad..........62
- Thai Grilled Sirloin Salad..........53

Salad Dressing
- French Salad Dressing..........72
- Italian Salad Dressing..........71
- Shrimp Dressing..........66
- Southwest Vinegar..........73
- Tomato-Herb..........74

Salmon, Poached..........136

Salsa
- Breakfast Burrito Salsa..........145
- Tomato Salsa..........102

Satay
- Chicken Satay..........117

Sauce
- Almond Sauce..........187
- Chocolate-Marshmallow Sauce..........187
- Egg Fu Yung Sauce..........147
- Marinara Sauce..........155
- Meat Sauce..........97
- Peanut Sauce..........118
- Piña Colada Sauce..........202
- Red Plum Sauce..........188
- Rum Sauce..........202
- Sweet and Sour Sauce..........105
- Soy Dipping Sauce..........159

Saucy Beef Noodles..........183
Sauerkraut and Pork Skillet..........87

Sausag
- Breakfast Burrito..........145
- Egg Casserole..........144
- Mardi-Gras Family Omelet..........143

Sauté, Asparagus Mushroom..........153

Scallop(s)
- Scallop Shrimp Jambalaya..........130
- Scallops with Chives and Peppers..........126

Scones, Griddle Oat..........166
Seafood File Gumbo..........138

Sesame
- Chinese Salad..........57
- Lemon Sesame Chicken..........109
- Sesame Chicken Wings..........79

Shells, Spinach Cheese Jumbo..........142
Shortcake, Stovetop Strawberry..........189

Shrimp
- Paella..........183
- Pasta Shrimp Salad..........176
- Pork and Shrimp Pot Stickers..........106
- Scallop Shrimp Jambalaya..........130
- Seafood File Gumbo..........138
- Shrimp Dressing..........66
- Shrimp Spring Rolls..........134

INDEX

Thai Red Curry Shrimp and Pineapple. 132

Singapore Fish…………………………... 139

Sirloin

    Thai Grilled Sirloin Salad…………… 53

Skillet

    Ground Beef Skillet Casserole……… 91

    Sauerkraut and Pork Skillet………… 87

    Skillet Cabbage……………………… 161

Soda Bread………………...………… 188

Soup

    Chickpea Soup w/Cumin & Cilantro… 51

    Chinese Beef-Noodle Soup………… 59

    French Onion Soup………………… 60

    Leeks, Mushroom and Potato Soup… 63

    Pinto Bean Soup…………………… 61

    Wedding Soup……………………… 56

Southwest Vinegar Dressing………………… 73

Soy Dipping Sauce…………………………… 159

Spices

    5-Spice Mix………………………… 204

    Blanched Almonds………………… 205

    Bouquet Garni……………………… 205

    Garam Masala…...………………… 204

    Indian Curry Spice Mix……………... 204

    Roasted Rice Powder……………… 205

    Tahini……………………………... 205

Spicy Carrots………………………………… 151

Spicy Wehani with Cashews…………………… 171

Spinach

    Spinach Cheese Jumbo Shells………… 142

    Spinach Fish Rolls…………………… 127

Spring Rolls

    Shrimp Spring Rolls………………… 134

    Vegetarian Spring Rolls……………… 158

Steak

    Marinated Flank Steak……………… 94

Steamed Mussels…………………...………… 131

Stew

    Blarney Stone Stew………………….. 93

    Pork and Pumpkin Stew…………….. 107

Stir Fry, Vegetable……………………………… 152

Stovetop Strawberry Shortcake………………… 189

Strawberry

    Fresh Strawberry Trifle……………… 190

    Frozen Strawberry Jam……………… 146

    Stovetop Strawberry Shortcake……… 189

    Strawberry Cheese Blintzes………….. 141

Stuffed Artichokes……………………………… 160

Stuffed Cabbage Rolls………...……………… 103

Stuffed Mushrooms…………………………... 76

Stuffed Peppers…………………...…………… 104

Stuffed Peppers, Ground Turkey………………... 119

Swedish Meatballs……………………………… 88

Sweet and Sour Pork………………...………… 105

Sweet and Sour Tuna………...………………… 137

Swiss, Meatballs a la…………………………… 89

Tahini…………………………………...…… 205

Teriyaki Chicken……………………………… 121

Thai Grilled Sirloin Salad…………………...…… 53

Thai Red Curry Shrimp and Pineapple…..……… 132

Thighs

    Chicken Thighs Marengo…………… 114

    Couscous with Chicken Thighs……… 172

Tikka, Chicken…………………………….... 116

Tomato

    Mussels in Tomato Broth…………… 131

    Tomato Salsa………………………… 102

    Tomato-Herb Dressing……………...… 74

Tortillas, Flour…………………………...… 100

Tossed Salad, Company…………………………… 70

Trifle, Fresh Strawberry……………………...…… 190

Tuna, Sweet and Sour ………………………...…… 137

Turkey

    Ground Turkey Stuffed Peppers……… 119

    Stuffed Cabbage Rolls……………… 103

    Turkey with Orzo and Broccoli……… 122

Upside-Down Cake

    Apricot Upside-Down Cake………… 196

    Pineapple Upside-Down Cake……… 195

Vegetable(s)

Asparagus Mushroom Sauté............ 153

Basmati Pea Pilaf......................... 168

Beef and Chinese Noodles.............. 76

Beef with Broccoli........................ 84

French Onion Soup....................... 60

German Potato Salad..................... 54

Green Beans and Fennel Salad.......... 68

Ground Turkey Stuffed Pepper.......... 119

Indian Cauliflower Salad................. 64

Leeks, Mushroom and Potato Soup...... 63

Orange Roughy a la Asparagus......... 125

Patata-Piccata Salad...................... 67

Pinto Bean Soup........................... 61

Potato Salad............................... 173

Roasted Pepper Salad.................... 62

Rosemary Potatoes....................... 156

Skillet Cabbage............................ 161

Sauerkraut and Pork Skillet.............. 87

Spicy Carrots.............................. 151

Spinach Cheese Jumbo Shells........... 142

Spinach Fish Rolls......................... 127

Stuffed Artichokes........................ 160

Stuffed Cabbage Rolls.................... 103

Stuffed Mushrooms....................... 76

Stuffed Peppers............................ 104

Turkey with Orzo and Broccoli.......... 66

Vegetable Curry........................... 157

Vegetable Stir Fry......................... 152

Vegetarian Spring Rolls.................. 158

Vinegar

    Southwest Vinegar Dressing.............. 73

    Tomato-Herb.............................. 74

Wedding Soup............................. 56

Wehani

    Spicy Wehani with Cashews............. 171

    Wings, Sesame

Chicken.................................... 79

Wrapped Chestnuts....................... 78

Yung, Egg Fu.............................. 147

R E S O U R C E S

The Surgeon General Report on Nutrition and Health, 1988 U.S. Department of Health and Human Service, Washington, D.C. 20402

Calorie Point Diet — a "point" in the right direction toward weight management, Still Regional Medical Center, Jefferson City, Missouri

Fit or Fat, Baily, Covert; Houton Mifflin Co., Boston, 1977

The Dieter's Dilemma, Bennet, William, M.D.; Gwin, Joel; Basic Books, Inc., New York, 1982

Exercise Physiology, McArdle, William D.; Katch, Frank I.; Victor L.; Lea and Febiger, Philadelphia, 1981

Fiber, Swartz, Roni, R.D.; Nutrition Information Center of Osteopathic Hospital, 2622 W. Central, Wichita, KS, 1983

Professional Guide to HCF Diets, James W. Anderson, M.D.; F.A.C.P. Beverling Sieling, R.D.; Wen-Ju Leu Chen, Ph.D.; Lexington, Kentucky, 1981, (Published by HCF Diabetes Research Foundation, Inc., 1872 Blaermore Rd., Lexington, Kentucky.)

Food Values of Portions Commonly Used, Jean A.T. Pennington and Helen Nichols Church, Harper & Row Publishers, New York, 13th Edition.

Wesley Calorie Point Book, Nutrition Department, HCS Wesley Medical Center, 550 N. Hillside, Wichita, Kansas

Made in the USA
Charleston, SC
19 June 2013